*Praise for* HUNDREDS OF HEADS™ *Su*

"Hundreds of Heads is an innovative publishing house...Its entertaining and informative 'How To Survive...' series takes a different approach to offering advice. Thousands of people around the nation were asked for their firsthand experiences and real-life tips in six of life's arenas. Think 'Chicken Soup' meets 'Zagats,' says a press release, and rightfully so."
—ALLEN O. PIERLEONI, "BETWEEN THE LINES," THE SACRAMENTO BEE

"At some point, the Chicken Soup for the Soul series has to run its course . . .Here's our contender for its replacement: The How to Survive series, published by Hundreds of Heads Books. Launched in 2004, the series flatly ignores 'experts' and offers funny but blunt advice from thousands across America who've walked some of life's rougher roads."
—LAURI GITHENS HATCH, ROCHESTER DEMOCRAT AND CHRONICLE

"The books have struck a nerve: Freshman Year was the No.1-selling college-life guide of 2004 . . ."
—TODD LEOPOLD, CNN.COM

"Hundreds of Heads Books hopes to make life in our complicated new millennium a bit more manageable...Rather than approach a handful of psychologists or other so-called experts, the editors have polled hundreds of 'real people' who have gone through the challenges and lived to tell about them."
—BILL ERVOLINO, "BOOKMARKS," THE RECORD, HACKENSACK, NEW JERSEY

"A concept that will be . . . a huge seller and a great help to people. I firmly believe that today's readers want sound bytes of information, not tomes. Your series will most definitely be the next 'Chicken Soup.'"
—CYNTHIA BRIAN
TV/RADIO PERSONALITY, BEST SELLING AUTHOR: CHICKEN SOUP FOR THE GARDENER'S SOUL; BE THE STAR YOU ARE!; THE BUSINESS OF SHOW BUSINESS

"Move over, 'Dummies'. . . Can that 'Chicken Soup!' Hundreds of Heads are on the march to your local bookstore!"
—ELIZABETH HOPKINS,
KFNX (PHOENIX) RADIO HOST, THINKING OUTSIDE THE BOX

"With warmth, humor and 'I've been there' compassion, editors Gluck and Rosenfeld have turned the ordinary experiences and struggles of parents into bits of compact wisdom that are easy to pick up and use straightaway. I especially liked this book's many examples of how to survive (and even thrive) while living under the same roof as your teen."

—JACLYNN MORRIS, M.ED.
CO-AUTHOR OF I'M RIGHT. YOU'RE WRONG. NOW WHAT? AND FROM ME TO YOU

"The book really gave me some insight on my life and hopefully my parents will read it so we can improve our relationship."

—DAVID E. WEINSTEIN
10TH GRADE CLASS PRESIDENT, RIVERWOOD HIGH SCHOOL
SANDY SPRINGS, GEORGIA

## HOW TO SURVIVE YOUR FRESHMAN YEAR

"This book proves that all of us are smarter than one of us."

—JOHN KATZMAN
FOUNDER AND CEO, PRINCETON REVIEW

"...a guide full of fantastic advice from hundreds of young scholars who've been there, as well as dropouts who reflect on their decision... It's a quick and fun read with short stories and quotes about the pros and cons of everything from getting a job during the school year to dating within your residence."

—BOSTON HERALD

"Voted in the Top 40 Young Adults books."

—PENNSYLVANIA SCHOOL LIBRARIANS ASSOCIATION

"Good advice about saying goodbye to your parents, dealing with homesickness, making new friends, and getting around campus. Should you live in a dorm or off campus? Oh, yeah, and what about studying? Alone or with groups? These questions and lots more (money, laundry, food, sex, parties, time-management, etc.) are addressed with honesty and humor. This would be a great book to have for the graduating high school seniors to make them less anxious about college."

—NORMA LILLY
M.L.S., INGRAM LIBRARY SERVICE, HIDDEN GEM

"This cool new book…helps new college students get a head start on having a great time and making the most of this new and exciting experience."

"Explains college to the clueless…This quick read is jam-packed with tidbits."

"This book is right on the money. I wish I had this before I started college."

## HOW TO SURVIVE DATING

"Rated one of the Top 10 Dating Books."

"Reading this book, I laughed out loud… I also decided to decree snippets a most superior art form for dating manuals."

"Whether you're single or not, *How to Survive Dating* will have you rolling with laughter…This isn't your ordinary dating book."

"Invaluable advice… If I had read this book before I made my movie, it would have been only *10 Dates*."

"Reading *How to Survive Dating* is like having a big circle of friends in one room offering their hard-earned advice about the toughest dating dilemmas. From the first kiss to knowing when it's time to say 'I love you,' this book can help you avoid the headaches and heartaches of dating. *How to Survive Dating* is a must-read for singles."

"Great, varied advice, in capsule form, from the people who should know—those who've dated and lived to tell the tale."

"'Be yourself' may be good dating advice, but finding Mr. or Ms. Right usually takes more than that. For those seeking more than the typical trite suggestions, *How to Survive Dating* has dating tips from average folks across the country. It's like having a few hundred friends on speed-dial."

—KNIGHT RIDDER/TRIBUNE NEWS SERVICE (KRT)

"Hilarious!"

—TEENA JONES
THE TEENA JONES SHOW, *KMSR-AM (DALLAS)*

## HOW TO SURVIVE A MOVE

"Hundreds of essential moving tips, real-life stories, and quotes by movers across the United States and Canada."

—LIBRARY JOURNAL

"As a realtor, I see the gamut of moving challenges. This book is great - covering everything from a 'heads-up' on the travails of moving to suggested solutions for the problems. AND... it's a great read!"

—JEANNE MOELLENDICK, RE/MAX SPECIALISTS, JACKSONVILLE, FLORIDA

*"How to Survive A Move* is full of common sense ideas and moving experiences from every-day people. I have been in the moving industry for 22 years and I was surprised at all the new ideas I learned from your book!"

—FRED WALLACE, PRESIDENT, ONE BIG MAN & ONE BIG TRUCK MOVING COMPANY

"Tidbits that are easy to digest when you're more concerned with packing boxes than spending hours reading a book."

—SAN DIEGO UNION-TRIBUNE

"The editors of *How to Survive A Move* went to the experts: average people who've been there and done that. Much of the advice is the kind you're unlikely to get from the experts—such as living east of where you work so you won't be driving into the sun, using T-shirts to pad breakable items, and making sure to pack, ahem, adult paraphernalia in a really, really well-sealed box."

—DEMOCRAT AND CHRONICLE (ROCHESTER, NEW YORK)

"Packed with some good moving advice."

"A good resource book for do-it-yourself movers to learn some of the best tips in making a move easier."

# HOW TO SURVIVE YOUR MARRIAGE

"Simple tricks to help save your marriage."

"I love this book!"

"A unique offering and sorely needed resource of advice/wisdom from men and women who have found creative solutions to the many challenges of marriage and now are reaping its awards."

*How to Survive Your Marriage* is a fun companion to research-based marriage manuals. Great for starting a discussion with your partner or laughing at the commonality of concerns that engaged couples often face."

"Reader-friendly and packed full of good advice. They should hand this out at the marriage license counter!"

"Full of honest advice from newlyweds and longtime couples. This book answers the question—'How do other people do it?'"

"This book is the best wedding present I received! It's great to go into a marriage armed with the advice of hundreds of people who have been through it all already."

# HOW TO SURVIVE YOUR BABY'S FIRST YEAR

"Both informative and entertaining, this book is an excellent resource and companion book to other books on babies and parenting."
—PARENTS & KIDS MAGAZINE

"What to read when you're reading the other baby books. The perfect companion for your first-year baby experience."
—SUSAN REINGOLD, M.A., EDUCATOR

"As a new parent, it helps to know that you're not alone in facing one of life's biggest challenges. *How to Survive Your Baby's First Year* offers a compilation of humorous quotes from mothers and fathers who survived parenthood."
—LOS ANGELES DAILY NEWS

"*How to Survive Your Baby's First Year*...offers tried-and-true methods of baby care and plenty of insight to the most fretted about parenting topics..."
—BOOKVIEWS

"An amazing kaleidoscope of insights into surviving parenthood, this book will reassure moms and dads that they are not alone in the often scary world of bringing up baby."
—JOSEF SOLOWAY, M.D., F.A.A.P.
CLINICAL ASSOCIATE PROFESSOR OF PEDIATRICS
WEILL MEDICAL COLLEGE OF CORNELL UNIVERSITY

"Full of real-life ideas and tips. If you love superb resource books for being the best parent you can be, you'll love *How to Survive Your Baby's First Year.*"
—ERIN BRWON CONROY, M.A.
AUTHOR, COLUMNIST, MOTHER OF TWELVE, AND CREATOR OF TOTALLYFITMOM.COM

"The Hundreds of Heads folks have done it again! Literally hundreds of moms and dads from all over offer their nuggets of wisdom—some sweet, some funny, all smart—on giving birth, coming home and bringing up baby."
—ANDREA SARVADY
AUTHOR OF BABY GAMI

# How
# to Lose
# 9,000 lbs.
# (or less)

# WARNING:

This guide contains differing opinions. Hundreds of heads will not always agree. Advice taken in combination may cause unwanted side effects. Use your head when selecting advice.

# How to Lose

Advice from **516** Dieters Who Did

# to Lose

# 9,000 lbs.

# (or less)

JOAN BUCHBINDER, MS, RD, LDN, FADA
AND JENNIFER BRIGHT REICH
SPECIAL EDITORS

**Hundreds of Heads Books, LLC**

ATLANTA

Illustrations © 2006 by Image Club
Large cover photograph by JupiterImages, Small cover photograph by PictureQuest

Library of Congress Cataloging-in-Publication Data
How to lose 9,000 pounds (or less): Advice from 516 dieters who did / Joan Buchbinder and Jennifer Bright Reich, special editors.
 p. cm. — (Hundreds of Heads survival guide series)
ISBN 0-9746292-8-6
 1. Weight loss.  2. Weight loss—Psychological aspects.
I. Buchbinder, Joan.  II. Reich, Jennifer Bright.  III. Series: Hundreds of Heads survival guide.
 RM222.2.H69 2006
 613.2'5—dc22
                                                                    2005021219

See pages 216-29 for credits and permissions.

NOTE: Advice contained in this book is not intended to be a substitute for the advice and counsel of your personal physician. Consult your physician before beginning any diet or exercise program. Advice contained herein does not reflect the views of HUNDREDS OF HEADS or the Special Editors.

Limit of Liability/Disclaimer of Warranty: Every effort has been made to accurately present the views expressed by the interviewees quoted herein. The publisher and editors regret any unintentional inaccuracies or omissions, and do not assume responsibility for the opinions of the respondents. Neither the publisher nor the authors of any of the stories herein shall be liable for any loss of profit or any other commercial damages, including but not limited to special, incidental, consequential, or other damages.

HUNDREDS OF HEADS™ books are available at special discounts when purchased in bulk for premiums or institutional or educational use. Excerpts and custom editions can be created for specific uses. For more information, please email sales@hundredsofheads.com or write to:

HUNDREDS OF HEADS BOOKS, LLC
#230
2221 Peachtree Road, Suite D
Atlanta, Georgia 30309

ISBN-10: 0-9746292-8-6
ISBN-13: 978-09746292-8-5

Printed in U.S.A.
10 9 8 7 6 5 4 3 2 1

# CONTENTS

# Introduction

At any given moment, more than one quarter of American men and one third of American women are on a diet. We spend $33 billion a year trying to lose weight. With all those people and all that money, you'd think we would be a nation of Twiggys. But a quick trip to the mall or a glance at the driver in the next car may convince you that most Americans are losing the battle of the bulge.

Yet there are plenty of people out there who have fought the fat fight and won. They have triumphed over our super-sized, more-is-better, couch-potato society. How did they do it? To find the secrets, our head-hunters went out and asked hundreds of people, triumphant veterans of the diet wars, who, having fought the good fight, stand taller—and thinner!—with wisdom to share.

Not every diet works and not every diet goal is reached; sometimes it's instructive to read what went wrong, and some of these stories are included here. While there is a lot of universality to the weight-loss struggle, there are plenty of unique, clever ideas out there. Our interviewers went out and talked to hundreds of people who have been fighting the weight-loss battle for days, months, and in some cases, years and decades. The best stories and advice we heard from all these dieters are included here. We offer hundreds of smart tips that worked for the folks in this book; they may well work for you, too. Why settle for advice from only one or two people? If two heads are better than one, as the saying goes, then hundreds of heads are even better.

Unless today is the first time you've ever thought of dropping a pound or two, you know that there are hundreds of diet books out there, many purporting to offer a 'quick fix' of one sort or another. This book is different: We don't claim to offer a recipe for instant salvation, but rather hard-won, down-to-earth advice from hundreds of people who found out the hard way what works and what doesn't, so that you can pick and choose from strategies that seem sensible and appropriate to you.

As you might expect, we heard opposing views on some topics: for every low-carb enthusiast, there's an equally dedicated low-fatter. You'll be able to read all points of view and choose for yourself. Think of this book as an all-you-can-eat, weight-loss-tip buffet!

JENNIFER BRIGHT REICH

The weight-loss industry in America is a multi-billion-dollar business, yet it is unregulated: Anyone can write a book espousing his or her philosophy on weight loss: low carb, low fat, high protein, food combining, or point systems, to name a few varieties. We let someone else tell us how much we should be hungry for, what we should be hungry for, and when we should be hungry for it. But there are many, many factors involved with weight loss, and it will never be as simple as whether or not your diet is low fat, high protein, or low carbohydrate.

When it comes to weight loss, there is a common expression that applies: "If you do what you've always done, you'll get what you've always gotten!" Do you keep going back on the same diet? Do you keep trying the most popular fad diet "du jour"? Do you return to the same diet clinic where you lost some weight while following their diet plan, but were never able to maintain the weight loss for long? Do you continue to repeat the same mistakes hoping for a different outcome. . . like buying a package of potato chips and telling yourself you will only eat a "small handful"? Unless you identify those behaviors that continue to sabotage your weight-loss efforts and replace them with realistic, acceptable, permanent behavioral and lifestyle changes, you will continue to get the results you have always gotten.

We hope that these weight-loss tips from others who have walked in your shoes inspire you to make even small and subtle changes to your weight-loss efforts. No one person's approach to weight loss works for every individual who is trying to lose weight. But selecting a handful of tips from the hundreds of dieters in this book is certain to help you in your weight-loss efforts. Remember, weight is a chronic condition, and whatever method you choose in order to lose weight, you'd better love it: you are going to have to do it for the rest of your life!

JOAN BUCHBINDER
CONSULTING NUTRITIONIST
MS, RD, LDN, FADA

# The Defining Moment: Why Lose Weight?

I t's your moment of truth. The time has come, and you're ready. Perhaps something has happened in your life—or is about to, such as a 10-year reunion or the upcoming wedding of a friend—that has caused you to commit once and for all to get in shape, lose weight, and look great. Don't waste another precious second. Let the transformation begin!

**I WAS SICK AND TIRED** of being sick and tired of disliking my body. You know when you have a bad hair day you walk around feeling a little "off" because your hair looks less than great? Having a body that looks less than great is like having a bad hair day every waking minute.

—CECE BLASE
ALAMEDA, CALIFORNIA
LBS. LOST 25

**TALK IS JUST TALK. THE FIRST POSITIVE STEP IS WHEN YOU PUT DOWN THE COOKIES.**

—ERIN DELEONIBUS
PITTSBURGH,
PENNSYLVANIA
LBS. LOST 35

**I** WEIGHED **189,** AT **5'2"!** I was so embarrassed that I wouldn't go anywhere, not even to visit relatives. I had always been a little person. Most of my life, I've weighed 100 to 105 pounds. But then I had some medical problems, and the weight just packed on. I hated myself so much that I used to stand in front of a mirror and cry and yell at myself.

—*DIANE SZYMANSKI*
*SOUTH BEND, INDIANA*
*LBS. LOST 72*

- - - - - - - -

**M**Y FRIEND ALWAYS TELLS the story of how her son got her started dieting when he was five by pointing to her belly and asking when his baby brother was going to come.

—*MARY WEBB*
*WHEELING, WEST VIRGINIA*
*LBS. LOST 15*

- - - - - - - -

**I** WAS GOING TO BE THE MAID OF HONOR at a friend's wedding. I knew that I didn't want to be the heaviest bridesmaid, so I started a major diet program right away. By the day of the wedding, I had lost so much weight that my bridesmaid dress was actually baggy.

—*JENNIFER*
*READING, PENNSYLVANIA*
*LBS. LOST 70*

- - - - - - - -

**I**F YOU ARE GETTING into your late twenties and you are starting to gain some weight, you have to put a stop to it right then and there. As you get into your thirties, it gets more and more difficult to take the weight off. Do it as young as you can.

—*C.M.*
*PITTSBURGH, PENNSYLVANIA*
*LBS. LOST 18*

## DIET DATA

Nearly two-thirds of adult Americans (about 127 million people) are over-weight or obese. Healthcare costs of American adults with obesity top $100 billion.

**OF COURSE I WANT TO LOSE WEIGHT,** because that is all society tells me to do. The clothes being sold these days barely fit women who have boobs or hips. Basically you're given no choice but to lose weight.

—*ALLY*
*BUFFALO GROVE, ILLINOIS*
*LBS. LOST 38*

. . . . . . . .

" My sophomore year in college I caught a fat joke from a friend and decided I'd had enough. "

—*MICHAEL KOURABAS*
*NEW YORK, NEW YORK*
*LBS. LOST 60*

. . . . . . . .

**I HAD A "MOMENT."** I got on the scale one morning and it flashed "299" at me. I was absolutely devastated and horrified. I couldn't believe that was me on that scale, and I felt that I would rather be dead than ever break 300.

—*ERICKA DUNHAM*
*SEATTLE, WASHINGTON*
*LBS. LOST 73*

. . . . . . . .

**I HAD A CLOSET FULL OF CLOTHES** that I couldn't wear, and I had taken to wearing my fiancé's jeans. But the defining moment for me was when I looked at a photo of myself that was taken on Christmas. I couldn't believe that I was that roly-poly: My head looked like a pumpkin!

—*JENNIFER K.*
*SHEBOYGAN, WISCONSIN*
*LBS. LOST 22*

**I gained the freshman 25, not 15!**

—*MIA KIRCHMEIER*
*REDMOND,*
*WASHINGTON*
*LBS. LOST 25*

# WHAT'S IN A WORD?

To many people the terms "overweight" and "obese" are interchangeable. In fact, they have distinct medical definitions.

The question of overweight vs. obese starts with Body Mass Index, or BMI, a simple mathematical formula that takes into account a person's height and weight in order to provide an estimate of the risk for weight-related diseases. Based on a simple calculation of height/weight$^2$, BMI thresholds are as follows:

| BMI | Considered |
| --- | --- |
| <=20 | Underweight |
| 20-24.9 | Ideal |
| 25-29.9 | Overweight |
| 30-39 | Obese |
| >=40 | Extremely Obese |

BMI does not measure body fat, and it is possible for two people with different body types to have the same BMI—for example, an athlete with a high percentage of muscle mass can have the same BMI as a person with a higher percentage of body fat if they have the same height and weight. Because of this, experts consider other factors, such as diet, level of physical activity, waist circumference, blood pressure, blood sugar, cholesterol, and family history of disease, when determining overall health.

There is a big difference between body weight and body composition. Body weight is how much you weigh when you step on a scale, including your bones, muscles, fat, water, organs, and clothes (if you're wearing them). Body composition refers to what that weight is comprised of, or what percentage of your total weight comes from fat, versus lean body mass (muscles, organs, bones, etc.).

Athletes may weigh more, or be heavier, or even overweight, because a larger percentage of their weight is derived from muscle mass. They may, however, have a very low percentage of their weight coming from fat, or adipose tissue; they are heavy but lean.

## PERCENT BODY FAT

|  | Males | Females |
|---|---|---|
| Minimum | 5% | 11% |
| Top Athletes | 7-11% | 12-18% |
| Ideal | 12-17% | 18-24% |
| Average | 18-21% | 25-28% |
| Obese | >25% | >30% |

# FEEL LIKE A MILLION BUCKS

I was the winner of the TV show *Joe Millionaire*, which aired a few years ago. It was a great experience, but there was one moment on the show that really reinforced what I already felt about my weight: Before the other 19 women and I arrived for the show, the producers asked for our clothing sizes. During the taping of the show, they sent all 20 of us into a room with a rack of dresses and told us each to select one gown. It was mayhem, and I couldn't find a dress that fit. I was the largest of the girls. Later, one of the other girls said, "Poor Zora, she is just a different shape and size." That very public moment just added to the feeling I'd had for years about my weight. The feeling of not being able to control my weight left me frustrated and disappointed. Practically a professional dieter, I had tried many different weight-loss programs and was desperate enough to try almost anything.

—Zora Andrich
Lambertville, New Jersey
lbs. lost 20

I WAS VERY ACTIVE IN SPORTS and have cartilage damage to both knees. It was so bad that if I did something physical, like dancing, the next day I had to elevate my legs so the swelling would go down. But now, after losing the weight, my knee pain is gone.

*KAREN PHILLIPS*
*LANSING, ILLINOIS*
*LBS. LOST 42*

* * * * * * * *

**"** I had goals that I wanted to achieve. One was to avoid having to take cholesterol medicine, and I did. The other was to be able to shop in the regular gals section, and now I can. **"**

—*SUSAN*
*ATLANTA, GEORGIA*
*LBS. LOST 40*

* * * * * * * *

BEING SUCCESSFUL IN LOSING WEIGHT is similar to being successful in kicking a smoking habit. I was a smoker for many years and even though I knew the habit was bad for me I did not, and could not, quit until I made up my mind that I wanted to quit—that I wanted to be healthy.

—*W.F.R.M.*
*OKLAHOMA CITY, OKLAHOMA*
*LBS. LOST 20*

I felt terrible. I had no energy, and I just felt uncomfortable in my own skin. I didn't want to feel that way for the rest of my life.

—*LARA LOEST*
*MILWAUKEE,*
*WISCONSIN*
*LBS. LOST 15*

**I HATE IT WHEN I GET OUT** of the shower and then I start sweating right away from the exertion. That's what motivates me, above everything else, to drop some pounds.

—*P.S.S.*
*CARNEGIE, PENNSYLVANIA*
*LBS. LOST 10*

• • • • • • • • •

**I HAD NEVER GONE TO A GYM** a day in my life until after my husband had heart surgery and he was forced to go. We did it together, and I joined to support him. I never thought a gym was for me, but after going for a year, I can't stop.

—*S.F.*
*BUFFALO GROVE, ILLINOIS*
*LBS. LOST 15*

• • • • • • • • •

**I'D BEEN UNHAPPY WITH MY APPEARANCE** for a couple of years, but despite gentle prodding from friends I'd always been able to rationalize my weight gain: I had a back injury, so I couldn't exercise. Then, one day when I was getting dressed, the rose-colored glasses suddenly came off. "Oh, my God!" I thought, staring into the mirror. "Look at that stomach and those hips!" I was absolutely mortified. That was the moment I realized things had to change.

—*E.C.*
*NEW YORK, NEW YORK*
*LBS. LOST 20*

# DIET DATA

Obesity increases your risk of developing conditions such as high blood pressure, type-2 diabetes, heart disease, stroke, gallbladder disease and cancer of the breast, prostate and colon. But even weight losses as small as 10 percent of your body weight can improve your health.

# CRUEL COMMENTS ABOUT WEIGHT

**MY FIVE-YEAR-OLD COUSIN SAID** "You used to be thin. What happened? You really got fat."

> —*LAURA BATOG*
> *FRANKLIN, MASSACHUSSETTS*
> *LBS. LOST 30*

●●●●●●●●●

**PEOPLE SAY,** "You have such a pretty face. Why don't you try to lose some weight?" It makes me want to strike them.

> —*LISA BOLIVAR*
> *TAMARAC, FLORIDA*
> *LBS. LOST 50*

●●●●●●●●●

**A FAMILY MEMBER** (who had consumed too much joy juice) said, "Jacquie, your ass is as wide as an ax handle." What did I do? I didn't speak to him for a week. What do I wish I had done? I wish I had not spoken to him for a year!

> —*JACQUIE MCTAGGART*
> *INDEPENDENCE, IOWA*
> *LBS. LOST 45*

●●●●●●●●●

**PEOPLE ARE QUICK TO MAKE COMMENTS LIKE,** "Should you be eating that?" No one asks an anorexic if she should be eating a sandwich!

> —*AMANDA VEGA*
> *SCOTTSDALE, ARIZONA*
> *LBS. LOST 40*

Last year, I was on vacation at the beach, and we took some pictures. I had previously been diagnosed with diabetes and sleep apnea, which are both obesity-related. But I still didn't realize how fat I was. It took seeing a picture of myself standing on a damn pier for me to realize that something had to change. If you suspect you need to lose weight, ask a friend or family member to take pictures when you're not expecting it: Cameras don't lie.

—Mark Scott
Safford, Arizona
LBS. LOST 50

• • • • • • • •

At school I was happily eating at Wendy's three times a week. It was an escape and something I enjoyed. Three months into the semester, I had gained 10 pounds. I didn't have love handles—I had rolls behind me and, out of nowhere, a gut that was larger than I had ever seen. I was like, "OK, I've gained weight. I'm fat now." It really hit me when I took our dog Gray for a walk. I used to be able to keep up with her, and all of a sudden, I was dragging. I thought, "This gut is serious bad news. I can't even move with this fat."

—C.B.
Franklin, Massachusetts
LBS. LOST 10-15

• • • • • • • •

## DIET DATA

Thirty percent of Americans identify themselves as overweight or obese; 64 percent really are overweight or obese.

For me, it was my husband's heart condition. Upon having heart bypass surgery several years ago, at the age of 45, my husband was put on a special diet and exercise regime. I found it much easier for my husband to stick to his diet if I also followed the low-fat, vegetable-rich eating plan.

—P. Leonard
Greenwood, Arkansas
LBS. LOST 20

# PREGNANCY POUNDS

**AFTER BEING PREGNANT FOR NINE MONTHS,** I just wanted to fit into my old clothes. The best feeling is to just get into your old clothes again.

> —*R.M.*
> *CAMBRIDGE, MASSACHUSETTS*
> *LBS. LOST 14*

• • • • • • • • •

**EXERCISE GOT ME WITHIN FIVE POUNDS** of my pre-birth weight, but the rest never came off until about three months after I quit nursing.

> —*L.G.*
> *ATLANTA, GEORGIA*
> *LBS. LOST 26*

• • • • • • • • •

**FOR THE FIRST FIVE MONTHS** after giving birth to twins, my weight gain was acceptable. My number one priority was taking care of the babies, and since I had to wake up in the middle of the night so often, I figured I deserved a cookie every time. Then the fog lifted from my eyes. Maybe it's because I'd finally caught up on my sleep by this point: who knows? I remember being in a store and trying on a size 14. I'd always been a size 8 before I got pregnant. This nagging voice in my head said, "From here, there's nowhere to go but a 16!" That was simply unacceptable. I knew it was time to change.

> —*JULIE MARTIN SUNICH*
> *TAMPA, FLORIDA*
> *LBS. LOST 53*

I realized I needed to lose weight when I couldn't fit into my pants any more.

—*David Feder*
*Des Moines, Iowa*
*lbs. lost 6*

**I'M STARTING TO GET THAT FAT** hanging down from my arms like my grandmother always had. That's what convinced me I absolutely had to diet. I don't want to look like my grandmother.

—*Peggy Wehr*
*Woodworth, Ohio*
*lbs. lost 6*

* * * * * * * *

**IN HIGH SCHOOL,** I trained myself to overeat. I was growing, and putting on pounds was good for all the sports I was involved in. I think it's a common problem among guys that we're used to eating until we are stuffed, and we're used to putting tons of junk in our bodies without seeing the effects. It will catch up to you as you get older and your metabolism slows down. At this point, you have to train yourself to eat more consciously.

—*Anonymous*
*San Francisco, California*
*lbs. lost 8*

* * * * * * * *

**MEN, STOP SUCKING YOUR GUT** in and let it hang out so you can see how big your belly really is. Stop trying to trick yourself and face facts: You need to diet.

—*Jennifer Maloe*
*Barrelville, Maryland*
*lbs. lost 11*

* * * * * * * *

**GET A PROFESSIONAL OPINION.** Go see your doctor. Maybe you are not overweight, but instead are being too tough on yourself. On the other hand, hearing that you need to change the way you live from someone whose opinion you respect—like a doctor—might spur you into action.

—*Jerry Rose*
*Cumberland, Maryland*
*lbs. lost 19*

**I NEED AN ANTI-GRAVITY SUIT** because gravity is doing a job on my body! It happens to everyone, but I'm not worried about everyone; I'm worried about me.

—*TAMMY NELSON*
*MIDLOTHIAN, MARYLAND*
*LBS. LOST 13*

❝❝ I went on a diet for health reasons. I'm overweight right now, and it gives me problems in my hips, knees and heels. ❞❞

—*KATHY MCCLINTIC*
*CENTENNIAL, COLORADO*
*LBS. LOST 30*

**I GOT PHOTOS BACK** from a trip to Maui: It was the first time I had seen a picture of myself on a beach in a long time. I couldn't believe how much weight I had gained in a matter of a few years; it was so depressing.

—*MARGARET STECK*
*SEATTLE, WASHINGTON*
*LBS. LOST 38*

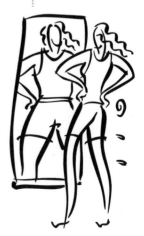

**I KNEW THAT I HAD TO DO** something about my weight once and for all after my oldest child went off to college. When I got home, I looked in the mirror and knew that it was time to take control of my life, beginning with my weight.

—*JOAN RAINWATER*
*WATERVILLE, OHIO*
*LBS. LOST 37*

# ONE THING I'D CHANGE ABOUT MY BODY

**MY LOVE HANDLES,** as my wife calls them: My wife tells me there's more of me to love, but I know she's just being nice.

> —M.B.
> CRANBERRY TOWNSHIP, PENNSYLVANIA
> LBS. LOST 18

• • • • • • • •

**MY FEET: THEY ARE FAT,** but no diet in the world is going to change that.

> —G.H.
> MOBILE, ALABAMA
> LBS. LOST 8

• • • • • • • •

**MY BEER GUT: WHEN I WAS YOUNGER,** I could drink and drink and never gain an ounce. Now all the beer I drink is sitting right here in my gut. I've tried to get rid of it but really haven't had any luck. Maybe I should stop drinking.

> —TODD CHARLESWORTH
> BOSTON, MASSACHUSETTS
> LBS. LOST 14

• • • • • • • •

**MY STOMACH:** Instead of a six-pack in my abdomen my wife says I have a keg there.

> —C.G.
> SALEM, OHIO
> LBS. LOST 11

• • • • • • • •

**MY DOUBLE CHINS:** I hate having them. I look in the mirror sometimes and wonder who the heck I am. I'm starting to look more and more like my dad. And that's scary.

> —LEROY BROWN
> BRADDOCK, PENNSYLVANIA
> LBS. LOST 41

**MY WHOLE BODY:** I wish I could change the way my body stores fat. I wish I could store it in the refrigerator, which is where most of the fat started out anyway.

> —*BILL DAVIS*
> *STRUTHERS, OHIO*
> LBS. LOST *2*

**MY GUT: I DON'T THINK** it would look so bad if I could distribute some of that weight to other parts of my body. Then it would look more even.

> —*REGGIE BONFIELD*
> *FROSTBURG, MARYLAND*
> LBS. LOST *8*

**MY THIGHS:** Even when I was a skinny little kid I had big fat thighs. And now that I'm heavy, they look like two tree trunks down there.

> —*JARED RHOADES*
> *MINNEAPOLIS, MINNESOTA*
> LBS. LOST *5*

**MY FINGERS:** They look like 10 little sausage links hanging off the end of my wrists.

> —*CHET YARO*
> *STRUTHERS, OHIO*
> LBS. LOST *8*

**MY ARMS. I SPENT A GOOD DEAL** of my younger years working out to build muscle, but now that I've let it go, it's turning to fat.

> —*E.H.*
> *SALEM, OHIO*
> LBS. LOST *12*

## DIET DATA

The heaviest man in history, Jon Brower Minnoch, weighed 1,399 pounds at his peak. On his diet he lost 923 pounds in 16 months.

**I KNEW IT WAS TIME TO DO** something about my weight when I had to hold my breath to tie my shoes while sitting down.

—*Tom*
*Kintnersville, Pennsylvania*
*lbs. lost 45*

• • • • • • • •

**I KNEW I NEEDED TO LIVE** a healthier lifestyle and lose weight after having a heart attack several years ago.

—*Michael Byrne*
*Gibbstown, New Jersey*
*lbs. lost 20*

# It's All in Your Head: How to Get–And Stay–Motivated

**N**ow the hard part begins. Anyone can start a diet, but here's how to stay motivated, day after dieting day. More important, here's how to dust yourself off and get back on the right track if you fall off the weight-loss wagon; even if you get run over by a Krispy Kreme truck.

I BOUGHT MYSELF A PAIR OF JEANS one size too small. Once a week I try them on. First I was able to just squeeze into them. Then I could pull them up. Finally I could zip them. Then I could actually put my hands in the pockets. Progress!

—MARY BRIGHT
ALLENTOWN, PENNSYLVANIA

SCREW THE REST OF THE WORLD; THIS IS ABOUT YOU.

—LISA BOLIVAR
TAMARAC, FLORIDA
LBS. LOST 50

Have a plan for yourself and stick to it. Don't procrastinate and say, "I'll start tomorrow," or "I can get away with this bad thing today."

—GRACE
CHAPEL HILL,
NORTH CAROLINA
LBS. LOST 15

## DIET DATA

If you burn 100 extra calories a day, you'll lose about 10 pounds in a year.

**IF YOU HAVE TROUBLE FINDING** motivation, look into the rates of heart disease of overweight people. Or look at the mortality rates. That'll give you some motivation.

—PAULA GRUBBS
RENFREW, PENNSYLVANIA
LBS. LOST 12

**MY 20-YEAR REUNION** crept up on me and before I knew it I had less than six months to lose all the weight my classmates had never seen on my skinny little frame. I didn't lose as much as I had hoped, but without the reunion I probably would not have bothered dieting at all.

—MARIA
EAST PALESTINE, OHIO
LBS. LOST 8

**A FRIEND SUGGESTED THAT** I join a boot camp. It was really beneficial. I was committing myself to a workout: I was focusing on getting in shape. The energy, just being there around people who wanted me to get into shape, people who were trained for that specific thing, was really motivational.

—C.B.
FRANKLIN, MASSACHUSETTS
LBS. LOST 10-15

**I WENT TO THE BANK** and got $100 in nickels: that weighs about 25 pounds. I put them in a backpack and took it everywhere I went. This helped me realize just how much extra weight I was carrying around every day and how much it was weighing me down. When I would lose a pound, I'd remove the equivalent weight in nickels.

—JEAN NICK
KINTNERSVILLE, PENNSYLVANIA
LBS. LOST 40

# THE WAKE-UP CALL

I wasn't feeling well, so I went to the doctor. After my exam, the doctor said, "What have you been doing to yourself? They are not going to give you a parade when you keel over. You are a mess. You need to do something about your health, or you are going to die." My blood sugar was out of control, and I was more than 99 pounds overweight. The doctor wanted to put me on insulin, but I said if he told me what to do, and what to avoid, that I would do it. The doctor's wake-up call was what I needed to hear to take the time to invest in myself. I lost the weight, went from a size 26 to a size 10 and never did need to go on insulin!

—JEANNIE LOFRANCO
SAN JOSE, CALIFORNIA
LBS. LOST 99

**I HAD A PAIR OF JEANS THAT** I hardly got to wear at all before I grew out of them. I made getting them back on the focus of the diet. I even hung them in my bedroom where I could see them every time I was in there.

—JOAN PIERSON
CRANBERRY TOWNSHIP, PENNSYLVANIA
LBS. LOST 15

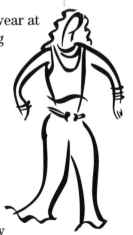

**WHAT MOTIVATES ME** is to sign up—and pay for—an exercise class. That increases my level of commitment: I'm forced to show up because I don't want to waste money!

—BETH W.
PHILADELPHIA, PENNSYLVANIA

# THE BEST TIME TO START A DIET

**WHEN YOU ARE READY TO MAKE** the commitment to change and stick with it.

> —*LISA BOLIVAR*
> *TAMARAC, FLORIDA*
> *LBS. LOST 50*

• • • • • • • •

**RIGHT BEFORE THE HOLIDAYS** instead of after: This way I had already created a new eating habit and didn't have to tell myself, "You'll diet after the first of the year."

> —*DANA LEAR*
> *LAWRENCEBURG, KENTUCKY*
> *LBS. LOST 125*

• • • • • • • •

**BETWEEN EASTER AND THE FOURTH OF JULY:** During the rest of the year, there are too many holidays and temptations to eat, and that gives me a good period of time with less temptation.

> —*SHELLEY*
> *PHILADELPHIA, PENNSYLVANIA*
> *LBS. LOST 43*

• • • • • • • •

**WHEN YOU ARE NOT STRESSED** out in other areas of your life! Don't try to move to a new state, start a new job, *and* go on a diet.

> —*LARA LOEST*
> *MILWAUKEE, WISCONSIN*
> *LBS. LOST 15*

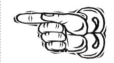

**YOU HAVE TO HAVE** a very specific goal to focus on: I mean, *extremely specific.* You have to think, "I want to lose 25 pounds by my high school reunion on June 11." Or, "I want to lower my cholesterol 10 points by my birthday." There's no such thing as too specific. For me it was my niece's wedding. I used that date as my goal to lose 20 pounds: I actually lost 22.

—A.P.
CORRIGANVILLE, MARYLAND
LBS. LOST 22

**"It's so much better to start with realistic goals that can be attained. If you set the bar too high, it will be difficult to maintain, and you'll get sick of it very quickly."**

—LISA A.
PHILADELPHIA, PENNSYLVANIA
LBS. LOST 20

**I'VE SET A REALISTIC GOAL** to lose an average of one pound a week, and then every two weeks I weigh myself to track my performance. I give myself a reward every 10 weeks only if my goal is met. Rewards: First, French manicure; second, spa pedicure; third, new red dress; fourth, leather jacket; fifth, complete new outfit, head-to-toe.

—V.B.
NEW YORK, NEW YORK
LBS. LOST 20

**LOSE WEIGHT TO SPITE ALL** the people who told you that you couldn't do it, or even all the people you suspect may have thought that, even if they didn't come right out and say it to your face. Do it to spite them all. Nobody ever said that you couldn't use spite as motivation, right?

—*GREG FOX*
*FROSTBURG, MARYLAND*
*LBS. LOST* **25**

**" As you get older it becomes harder to stay in shape. But the good news is that it happens to everyone. At your 25-year high school reunion, you'll see what I mean. "**

—*ANONYMOUS*
*NEW YORK, NEW YORK*
*LBS. LOST* **20**

**IF YOU'RE A PARENT,** you shouldn't need any motivation other than wanting to be healthy for your children. You should want to live a long life for them and be healthy enough that you can do stuff with them. I know how proud my kids are of how far I have come. I can see it in their eyes.

—*EVELYN RHODES*
*CAMPBELL, OHIO*
*LBS. LOST* **17**

# THE WORST TIME TO START A DIET

**AT THE BEGINNING OF THE COLD WEATHER.** Your body is gearing up for winter; it's natural to gain a few pounds then, which will make you feel like a failure. It's better to start at the beginning of spring. You have the motivation of summer clothes that you want to wear, and good fruits and veggies are coming into season. With that warm summer breeze coming in the door, it's easy to want to live on smoothies and salads, but not in November when everyone's tempting you with pumpkin pie!

> —*BRENDA*
> *CHARLESTON, WEST VIRGINIA*
> *LBS. LOST 25*

**DURING ANY STRESSFUL PERIOD OF TIME** or change; if someone is sick or if I have a big occasion coming up in my life.

> —*MICHELLE*
> *BIRMINGHAM, ALABAMA*
> *LBS. LOST 30*

**JUST BEFORE MY MENSTRUAL CYCLE:** all I crave is chocolate, salt, and everything else you probably shouldn't eat.

> —*SHELLEY*
> *PHILADELPHIA, PENNSYLVANIA*
> *LBS. LOST 43*

# THE POWER OF *YOU*: DIETING TIPS

*Self-efficacy, or the belief that you can modify your own behavior through willpower, is essential to permanent weight loss. Studies, including one from the* Journal of the American Dietetic Association, *show that increased self-efficacy leads to an increase in weight lost. Here are some tips:*

**TALK TO YOURSELF:** Create affirmations—positive statements about yourself that remind you of your desirable attributes. Use these to replace your negative thoughts about yourself. For example: Instead of focusing on the size of your stomach, remind yourself every day, "I have great looking legs!"

**FAILURE ISN'T FATAL:** Just because your last diet didn't last doesn't mean that this one won't, and thinking negatively can lower your confidence. More than 90 percent of people who have lost weight permanently failed at least once in losing and keeping off the pounds. To be truly successful you must walk around with a completely positive attitude that you will lose weight. Weight loss is too difficult to afford any pessimism.

**KEEP INSPIRED:** Think about times when you succeeded at something challenging. Compare the way that you overcame the odds that time with your current struggles. For example: If you are able to go out to dinner, and have one piece of bread (not three), order a filet mignon (instead of a porterhouse) with a baked potato topped with sour cream (instead of fried potato strings), then you have done a great job of staying focused on your weight-loss goals while still enjoying life.

**SET SMALL GOALS:** Seeing results right away will boost your confidence and keep you motivated. Small goals are an easy way to help yourself believe that you can achieve anything. For example: When trying to cut the calories from drinking two glasses of wine every night, don't say you'll never drink alcohol again; start by refraining from having a drink for two days out of seven.

**PREPARE FOR THE WORST:** Think about how you'll deal with roadblocks you may encounter on the way to reaching your goals before you get to them, so that if something comes up, you'll already have a plan to deal with it. For example: If you are going to a summer barbecue, simply tell yourself before you get there that you will abstain from the other temptations that aren't so important to you, like the chips and dips. Along with your hot dog, have corn on the cob, watermelon, and cherries, and enjoy the hot dog with no guilt!

**GET SUPPORT:** The people around us have an enormous impact on the way we view ourselves and on our ability to succeed. Role models can help you see the viability of your goals, and supportive friends and family members can help keep your confidence high. For example: Talk to your friends and family members who have been successful with their weight-loss efforts not just by losing weight, but by demonstrating that they can keep the weight off. If they can do it, so can you.

**BE HONEST WITH YOURSELF:** Make sure that you hold yourself accountable for your successes and your failures. This will make you feel in control and empowered, even when things aren't going well, and when they are, you'll be all the prouder knowing that you're responsible. For example: If you overeat on a Saturday night, wake up Sunday morning, and tell yourself you will get back on track today; do not wait for magical Monday to resume your weight-loss efforts. A lapse is not a collapse!

**BE INFORMED:** Educating yourself about what you're doing gives you a clearer idea of your goals and the obstacles you face. That way, you can be in control of the situation at all times. For example: consider a consultation with a Registered Dietitian or other qualified professional in the area of weight control, to help you critique your eating styles and nutritional needs.

**SEX IS THE BEST MOTIVATION:** It makes you want to be fit and helps you stay fit!

—*J.P.*
*NEW YORK, NEW YORK*

• • • • • • • •

" Find a fairly recent picture of yourself when you were looking mighty fine and put it in a prominent place. Visualization helps: Hey, you looked good once, you can do it again! "

—*STEPHEN MACKAY*
*SAN FRANCISCO, CALIFORNIA*
*LBS. LOST 10*

• • • • • • • •

**MY MOTIVATION WAS PRETTY** simple: to extend my life.

—*PAULINE T. MAYER*
*SMITHTOWN, NEW YORK*
*LBS. LOST 35*

# A KICK-START

If you've stopped losing weight after a promising start, you probably need to exercise a little harder than before. Any little changes will help kick-start your diet again, like adding resistance, doing more repetitions, and keeping it up longer.

# GET HELP.COM

**THE FIRST THREE WEEKS** on my restricted diet, I was going crazy! I was cranky and frustrated. I learned online that some of that was due to withdrawal symptoms and the other was a bitterness that I couldn't enjoy some foods I loved! There are so many diet communities that are easy to access, and I have found very supportive and insightful people. I can get questions answered and also learn good tips on how to prepare foods I can eat.

> —*MICHELLE*
> *TORONTO, ONTARIO, CANADA*
> *LBS. LOST 15*

• • • • • • • •

**I FOUND CALORIESCOUNT.COM,** a program that stresses healthy eating and exercise for life. It offers calculators to figure out how many calories are in foods, logs to keep track of the number of calories you eat, recipes, and meal plans. But more important, it offers message boards where I went often to talk with people in the same situation I was in, and to ask for advice. The program gave me both the resources and the support I needed. Even 13 months after losing the weight, I still check in a few times a week.

> —*JOAN RAINWATER*
> *WATERVILLE, OHIO*
> *LBS. LOST 37*

• • • • • • • •

**I GO TO A WEB SITE CALLED OBESITYHELP.COM.** It's a wonderful support group for people in every stage of the weight-loss process. Best of all, it's free!

> —*BONNIE SMITH*
> *MANCHESTER, MISSOURI*
> *LBS. LOST 100*

**DIET DATA**
If you're moderately obese, your life expectancy could be shortened by two to five years.

I only diet for beauty reasons, and if I get healthy along the way, that is a great bonus.

—V.B.
NEW YORK,
NEW YORK
LBS. LOST 20

**COMMIT TO DIETING ONLY** when you feel it is imperative: before a wedding or reunion, the week after the holiday season, or when you just want to lose those last five pounds that have been keeping you from feeling stunning! Start early, give yourself at least two weeks to see results, and don't expect it to fall off overnight.

—M.J.F.
NEW YORK, NEW YORK
LBS. LOST 5-10

• • • • • • • • •

**DON'T BE DESPERATE** to change yourself overnight. After I had to buy clothes a size larger than I always had been, I was determined to graduate from college weighing close to what I was when I started college. This would mean losing about 15 pounds over the course of a few months. I achieved that goal, and then continued with eating better, eating less, and exercising a little more.

—K.H.
NORMAN, OKLAHOMA
LBS. LOST 45

• • • • • • • • •

**DON'T GIVE YOURSELF** short-term goals (for instance, looking hot for a party in three weeks), but focus on long-term goals. Otherwise, you will diet like crazy until the event date and then let it all go.

—F.V.
NEW YORK, NEW YORK
LBS. LOST 15

• • • • • • • • •

**TAPE A PICTURE OF YOURSELF** to the refrigerator as motivation. Every time you go to the refrigerator you'll think twice about what you're doing.

—CHERI HURD
LITTLETON, COLORADO
LBS. LOST 30

**NEXT SUMMER WE ARE GOING** to Greece, where my mother's family is from. The airline tickets have been bought and the hotel reservations have been made, but I told my mom I'm not going unless I lose 15 pounds. I don't want my long-lost relatives' first impression of me to be that I am just another overweight American. My mom is holding my ticket and I have made her promise me that she will not allow me to go unless I lose the weight.

—*BESSIE SARVER*
*BAZETTA, OHIO*
LBS. LOST *10*

" Weight loss boils down to a lot of hard work, willpower, and commitment. And no matter what plan or diet you follow, without those three things nothing is going to work. "

—*KANDI KIZZIAH*
*ROCKY MOUNT, NORTH CAROLINA*
LBS. LOST *158*

**IT'S THE LITTLE THINGS** that add up to weight loss. Think of it as a series of small battles: Walk, don't ride; take the stairs, not the elevator; single cheeseburger instead of double; one shot of whiskey instead of two.

—*SANDY J.*
*ZELIENOPLE, PENNSYLVANIA*
LBS. LOST *24*

# WHAT WOULD POOH DO?

I wait to diet until the winter, because I can store my food and shoes in the trunk of my car. The food doesn't perish, and I have to really want it to go out for it. The cutest part of my diet was running out in the late morning for a bit of cereal. I'd look both ways first in the alley where my car would be parked, trying to gauge if I could make it to and from the house without anyone seeing me. Most days I did. But there were moments where I was caught on someone's mental candid camera—barefoot, with bed head, toting a box of Fiber One, and hovering around a 1988 Jetta with the trunk up, eating like a bear in a campsite.

—SHANNON
SEATTLE, WASHINGTON
LBS. LOST 15

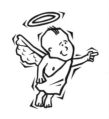

WE'RE ALL GOOD AT RATIONALIZING when we're on a diet, so rationalize backwards: Talk yourself into good behavior. Instead of "Well, if I just have one cookie, it won't hurt," tell yourself "Well, one cookie will taste good for 30 seconds, but my abs will look great in that bikini all summer," "If I only have half of this pasta, my pants will zip without me holding my breath," etc. Sucker yourself into following your plan.

—ANONYMOUS
BOSTON, MASSACHUSETTS

• • • • • • • • •

MY MOTIVATION WAS ALL THE PEOPLE, including my doctor and my ex-husband, of all people, who said I'd never lose the 20 extra pounds I gained while I was pregnant with my son. I knew I could do it if I stuck to it.

—B.V.
NORTH JACKSON, OHIO
LBS. LOST 19

AFTER I DECIDED I HAD TO LOSE the weight, I lost
12 pounds the first month. That's when I realized
I could lose 100 pounds in a year, two pounds per
week. I weighed in every single Sunday and kept
track of my weight on a chart. It wasn't easy, but
by being rigid and militant with my diet, I lost
two pounds almost every single week. Once you
make up your mind about something, you can do
anything.

—*KARA*
*CHICAGO, ILLINOIS*
*LBS. LOST 217*

. . . . . . . .

" I recently decided to lose weight
before my 30th birthday. I have
a sign on my treadmill that
reads, '30 by 30.' I'm
optimistic. "

—*ANONYMOUS*
*BIRMINGHAM, ALABAMA*
*LBS. LOST 30*

. . . . . . . .

FULL-LENGTH MIRRORS ARE EXCELLENT motivators.
So is the TV. Media images provide constant pres-
sure to get fit, lose weight, and develop 12-pack
abs. For guys, there's pressure to look like Brad
Pitt; for girls, there's pressure to look like Mary-
Kate Olsen. Ironically, the same medium that
feeds us these images also assaults us with
McDonald's ads, so it's a confusing scenario.

—*J.A.*
*IOWA CITY, IOWA*
*LBS. LOST 15*

**DIET DATA**
While men are
more likely to
be over-
weight than
women,
women are
more likely
than men to
be obese.

Simple changes got me started. For example, when I started my diet, I resolved not to eat anything after 9 p.m., and I switched to fat-free foods.

—*Molly Brown*
  *Allentown,*
  *Pennsylvania*

**My sorority sister buys jeans** a size too small and hangs them on her wall for constant motivation. I guess this really works; she's eventually able to fit into them.

—*Kristen Hurd*
  *Tulsa, Oklahoma*
  *lbs. lost 20*

• • • • • • • •

**It's important to be realistic** and flexible about your goals. Everyone is different. A weight chart might say that if you are 4′11″ you should weigh 85 pounds, but that's just a standard. Set goals that make sense for you. I'm 4′11″ but I'm built like Mary Lou Retton: I'm never going to weigh 85 pounds.

—*Amanda Vega*
  *Scottsdale, Arizona*
  *lbs. lost 40*

# High Visibility or Homegrown: Brand-Name and Other Dieting Options

*Millions of Americans have tried the brand-name weight-loss plans with some rate of success. And, while the diet industry has programs and books galore, plenty of clever people came up with their own dieting strategies and programs that worked.*

LOSING WEIGHT IS A SIMPLE MATTER of mathematics. You have to burn off more calories than you take in each day; that's it. Eat sensibly and exercise, and the weight will come off.

—CHRISTINE MCCARTHY
PORT ZELIENOPLE, PENNSYLVANIA
LBS. LOST 10

REMOVE THESE TWO WORDS FROM YOUR VOCABULARY: SUPER AND SIZE

—KARA DEPASQUALE
PITTSBURGH, PENNSYLVANIA
LBS. LOST 15

**I KNOW LOW CARB WORKS** for me, but it's difficult not to eat carbs, especially bread. So, instead, I eat bread in moderation and try to focus on cutting out desserts as much as possible. This works just as well.

—*L.A.*
*CLEVELAND, OHIO*
*LBS. LOST 8*

* * * * * * * *

**"Find out how expensive certain diet plans are before you start one. My wife tried Optifast, and it cost about $700 a month for all the proper food and pills."**

—*RANDY FREITIK*
*PEORIA, ILLINOIS*

## OUTSMARTED

If your body detects any major drop in calorie intake, your metabolism will adjust itself by burning fewer calories a day.

* * * * * * * *

**ALWAYS BE ON THE LOOKOUT** for a new diet. I have been on every diet under the sun, and they always work great the first time but not the second. I lost 20 pounds through hypnosis, but the second time I didn't pay enough attention. I lost 10 pounds through acupuncture, but the second time my body ignored the needle jolts. I tried eating low carb, which worked well, but by the second attempt, my body was not fooled; it knew the carbs would be back soon.

—*S.C.*
*SAN ANTONIO, TEXAS*
*LBS. LOST 10*

# DEEP STUFF

I'm 55 years old, and I've been on some kind of diet for about 24 years. Have they worked? Yes; briefly. But the one I have been on for several years really works: Overeater's Anonymous. Sure, counting calories and watching what you eat makes those of us who are overweight lose weight—fast. But the bottom line is that I overeat for one reason: Food gives me comfort. Not cozy comfort, but comfort that I'm preventing myself from becoming who I really want to be—a fit, attractive, healthy person. That's the deep stuff that O.A. is all about.

Based on the model of A.A., it deals with food as an addiction. Unlike A.A., you can't give up food like alcohol, but you can and must stick to a plan of moderation, and benefit from a nonjudgmental support network. The big questions you work on are: What demons are driving you to eat much more than you need? What comfort does food give you that you can find elsewhere? What makes you afraid about being attractive? If you really want to lose weight, you'd better figure those questions out.

—*Anonymous*
*Alford, Massachusetts*

# WHAT THEY SAY ABOUT ...

*Millions of Americans have tried Weight Watchers. Here are what some of our respondents had to say about the program.*

**I DID WEIGHT WATCHERS FOR ABOUT THREE MONTHS,** and it was a love-hate relationship. I loved the results (lost 14 pounds in the first month and a half), but I hated writing down everything I ate and calculating each food I was consuming.

> —*DEANNA*
> *LIBERTYVILLE, ILLINOIS*

**WEIGHT WATCHERS WORKS.** Like the commercial says: It's about real food and learning how to balance it out—portions, ingredients, and frequency. Also, having the weigh-in each week was helpful. I rarely stay for the meeting portion; it's enough motivation to see the others, chat briefly, and move on.

> —*ANONYMOUS*
> *LOS ANGELES, CALIFORNIA*
> *LBS. LOST 20*

**I LOST WEIGHT WITH WEIGHT WATCHERS,** the online version. I'm not really a sit-around-and-talk-about-your-cravings-with-strangers kind of gal, so I did the online thing and it worked great.

> —*KIM N.*
> *MT. LAUREL, NEW JERSEY*
> *LBS. LOST 45*

**I HAVE AN INCREDIBLE, INSPIRING GROUP LEADER.** Seeing her each week is a little like going to church: I feel all revved up and full of fresh resolve afterwards.

> —*CECE BLASE*
> *ALAMEDA, CALIFORNIA*
> *LBS. LOST 25*

**THE KEY TO DIETING SEEMS** to be the key to all things in life: moderation. This means cutting down the size of all meals and snacks. In the first phases of it, I also cut out all sweets. For about six months, I wouldn't eat candy, cookies, cake, ice cream, anything of that nature. Unfortunately I inherited a major sweet tooth from my father, so this was a difficult process. Now, almost three years since I dropped the weight, I still eat in moderation, but I can eat whatever I want.

—*MICHAEL KOURABAS*
*NEW YORK, NEW YORK*
*LBS. LOST 60*

"Get a diet buddy—someone who will call when you don't show up for your Weight Watchers meeting and make you go for a walk when you confess to polishing off the brownies."

—*NATALIE GROSDAYK*
*JAMAICA ESTATES, NEW YORK*
*LBS. LOST 12*

**FOR ME, ONE OF THE KEYS** to surviving the low-carb way of eating is to realize that this is not a diet; it's a way of life. I've never felt better, looked better, or been in better health.

—*CAROL R.*
*PHILADELPHIA, PENNSYLVANIA*
*LBS. LOST 38*

I'm on the Toddler Diet: You don't get to eat sitting down, and you don't get seconds.

—LISA BARNSTROM
SAN ANTONIO,
TEXAS
LBS. LOST 40

**IF YOU MUST DIET, DO IT SENSIBLY.** No crazy, trendy diets (i.e., liquid, grapefruit, or any plan that limits your calories to less than 1,000 a day), or else you are setting yourself up to gain back whatever weight you may lose. Not into dieting? No problem. Just eat well-balanced meals most days and exercise like crazy!

—G.N.
FT. SMITH, ARKANSAS
LBS. LOST 15

• • • • • • • •

**FIRST I DECIDED HOW MUCH** I wanted to lose each month. Then I made a chart, an actual graph that showed how much I weighed and how much I wanted to weigh. I drew a diagonal line from one point to the other, then I marked off the calendar days. I weighed myself at exactly the same time each day. The object was to hit the weight designated for each day. If my weight was above the line on the chart I ate 400 calories less that day and increased my exercise. If I weighed a couple of pounds below the day's target, I'd allow myself a little treat. There was something compelling about that magic line on the chart; the weight just melted off.

—ANONYMOUS
DES MOINES, IOWA

# MY OWN DIET

In spite of all of the branded diets on the market, the most popular diet plan in America is the one a dieter creates for himself. Twenty-five percent of Americans have made up their own diets, and at any given time seven percent of us are on one.

**START COOKING FOR YOURSELF,** especially if you're used to eating a lot of fast food. There's no way you can cram as much fat and salt into a home-cooked meal as you get in fast food: well, maybe you could, but you'd have to be trying really hard.

—*FRED*
*WASHINGTON, D.C.*
*LBS. LOST 17*

. . . . . . . .

" Eat real, fresh food that happens to be naturally low in whatever you are avoiding. Your body will thank you for eating real blueberries instead of blueberry fruit spread product with fake sugar and soy-derived thickener in it. "

—*APRIL SMITH*
*BOSTON, MASSACHUSETTS*

. . . . . . . .

**THE DIET THAT I'VE FOUND** works best for me is simple: Cut out the sugar. I was eating so much sugar on a daily basis without really realizing it. Making little changes—like not using syrup on my pancakes and not eating desserts but a hand-ful of nuts instead—has made a huge difference!

—*ANONYMOUS*
*NEW YORK, NEW YORK*
*LBS. LOST 20*

# PUT IT IN WRITING

**KEEP A JOURNAL OF YOUR DAILY EATING HABITS.** On the first page, list your ideal diet in terms of types of foods and servings. For each day of the diet, record everything you intake orally (even down to those glasses of water and tiny pieces of candy). At the end of each day, tally up the types of food you ate according to the Food Guide Pyramid (carbohydrates, fruits, vegetables, dairy, meat, fats, oils, sweets) and also water intake. It's an amazing wake-up call since it shows you what you are really putting into your body each day. You will be able to see if you are neglecting a food group or overcompensating with another.

—*BETHANY AMBROSE*
*BETHESDA, MARYLAND*
*LBS. LOST 5*

*. . . . . . . . .*

**WRITE DOWN EVERYTHING THAT YOU EAT.** This has helped me stick to my 1,500-calorie-a-day diet. You can eat a lot for 1,500 calories if you eat fruits, vegetables, and lean protein. One trip to a fast-food restaurant, though, and you're done for the day.

—*TRUDY*
*SPRINGVILLE, UTAH*
*LBS. LOST 8*

*. . . . . . . . .*

**I COUNTED CALORIES, PLAIN AND SIMPLE.** The advice came from my mother, who is 5'4" and lost 40 pounds this way! I kept a journal recording the calorie content of everything—every single snack, everything—that I ate for about a month. I worked on it until I was down to around 1,300 calories a day. I also walked two miles a day. I lost five pounds almost immediately.

—*NAOMI*
*SAN FRANCISCO, CALIFORNIA*
*LBS. LOST 8*

**I WENT LOW-CARB BECAUSE** the foods that cause me to overeat are mostly sugars and breads. I figured eliminating them would be the best way to go. However, I wasn't as strict as some people. I love salads, so I allowed myself lettuce and vegetables. As well, I ate jelly beans, Reese's Peanut Butter Cups and other sweets made with Splenda (a sugar substitute). I lost weight slowly, which was OK. I've been able to keep it off because I took the parameters of a successful diet program and personalized them for me.

—*JULIE MARTIN SUNICH*
*TAMPA, FLORIDA*
*LBS. LOST 53*

"Try meditation. Every night I sit in my quiet office and visualize myself thinner. Initially I saw myself as a size 10, then an 8, then a 6. It was extremely helpful for me."

—*PAULINE T. MAYER*
*SMITHTOWN, NEW YORK*
*LBS. LOST 35*

**IT DOESN'T MATTER** who endorses a certain diet or what kind of average weight loss it claims. Talk it over with your doctor to be sure whatever you do is right for you.

—*HELEN HUGHES*
*CLEVELAND, OHIO*
*LBS. LOST 35*

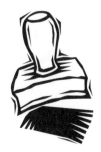

# GOOD CARBS/BAD CARBS

Our muscles are fueled from the energy in carbohydrates. Unfortunately, carbohydrates have received some bad press of late. But not all carbohydrates are the same. Fruits and vegetables are the healthiest of all carbohydrates and contribute the fewest total calories of any food. They are filled with antioxidants and phytochemicals, which are substances that help to protect against heart disease and cancer. The more colorful the fruit or vegetable, the greater the health benefits. There are starchy or complex carbohydrates such as breads, bagels, English muffins, pasta, rice, and cereal. They are generally healthy foods—until we load them with high-fat toppings. Fiber is an indigestible form of carbohydrate. It is essential for ridding the body of carcinogens and cholesterol. And there is a form of carbohydrate called simple sugar, found in cookies, cakes, candy, soda, muffins, donuts, ice cream, etc. To lose weight, most health professionals will recommend reducing these empty-calorie sources of refined sugars.

**DRINK A TON OF WATER** and watch your portions. Portion size can be a hard thing to learn. Before, I would pour a bunch of cereal in a bowl. Now I measure it in my two-third-cup measurer and use a small cereal bowl so the amount looks bigger.

—LEESA
REDMOND, WASHINGTON
LBS. LOST 27

**YOU WANT A DIET WHERE** you're getting enough protein. People who are not informed eat a lot of vegetables, but they don't get enough protein. For me, one serving of protein is about the size of the palm of my hand. You should find out what good protein is. And make sure you eat every four to five hours—three meals with that much protein and some vegetables, and two small snacks between meals.

—C.G.
*RIDGEFIELD, CONNECTICUT*
*LBS. LOST 10*

• • • • • • • •

**AFTER I JOINED A WEIGHT-LOSS** support group at work, I lost weight initially but then my weight got stuck. I became very frustrated and discouraged. I talked with a personal trainer about my diet. I'm Chinese, and I eat a lot of rice, so he suggested cutting down on all of those carbs gradually. I cut my rice portions slowly, by about a tablespoon a week, and started eating more vegetables. It worked!

—*LORETTA*
*OREM, UTAH*
*LBS. LOST 15*

Being a vegetarian certainly doesn't make you skinny. There are plenty of cakes, cookies, and candies that fit a vegetarian diet.

—*ANONYMOUS*
*MERRICK,*
*NEW YORK*

# SLIM STATS

More than half of Americans surveyed say, "I eat whatever tastes good to me." But 23 percent say they monitor the nutritional value of what they eat, 17 percent follow a low-fat or low-sugar diet, and 15 percent follow a low-carb diet.

# REPORT FROM THE DIETING FRONT

*He's been there, he's done it, and he's here to tell you how it was.*

**FASTING**—A desperation tactic, and it works, especially when you're younger, but after you lose the weight that you want with any diet, there's always the "I was such a stud with that effort that I deserve a break" phase that sometimes has no endpoint. It's the worst with fasting, because you think that you deserve to eat more, post-diet, because you suffered so much. So a few months later, sometimes sooner, you gain all the weight back and more.

**HIGH-PROTEIN DIET**—Works wonderfully but has terrible effects. Heredity aside, I think this diet tickled gout and other afflictions, like hypertension and kidney stones, out of dormancy and into my life, like evil being unleashed from a sealed tomb in a B-movie. Weight does come off relatively quickly with a high protein diet, but if you have a crystal ball that shows your health in five, ten, fifteen years, you would think twice. The high-protein way is just not worth the inevitable pain and aggravation.

**HAND-HOLD DIET**—You go to a legitimate weight-loss clinic where you're assigned a nutritionist who designs a program for you and meets with you weekly. You're also weighed on some elaborate scale that can tell you your body mass index and all sorts of things you don't want to know. The physician on staff can help you with medications when it is medically appropriate, but thankfully I didn't have to go that route. But the lower calorie regimen and the weekly monitoring/counseling was miraculously effective. Three years ago I took part in the program for six months and the lifestyle change has stuck with me. The weight still fluctuates—it's now on the high side—depending on how rigidly I stick to the program, but I truly know what I need to do to get results. In the past, I simply looked for another diet.

**BODY FOR LIFE**—Ultimately failed me because the diet allows one free day per week that allows you to eat anything you want. On the first free day, I bought a Boston cream pie from a bakery, took it home, and ate it. On the next free day, I bought two Boston cream pies. The next free day, three Boston cream pies; you get the picture. This diet, in my case anyway, diminished brain capacity.

—*EDGAR POMA*
*SAN FRANCISCO, CALIFORNIA*
*LBS. LOST 30*

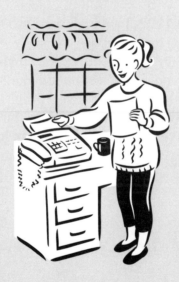

**I follow what I call the Easy Diet: I cut out fatty foods (like fried foods, dairy, and red meat): it's quite cheap and practical to do.**

—*MITCH G.*
*LOS ANGELES,*
*CALIFORNIA*

**I DEVELOPED IRRITABLE BOWEL SYNDROME** (IBS). What cured it was a revolution in my diet: I don't eat any processed foods, fast foods, or packaged foods, because our bodies weren't designed to eat those things. I eat a lot of nuts, fruits, and vegetables. I do eat protein; I'm not a vegetarian, but I don't eat a lot of red meat. As a result I am so much healthier. And I don't even think about dieting; I don't have to, because the way I eat now, I simply don't gain weight. I lost 40 pounds in less than three years.

—*D.W.*
*SAN DIEGO, CALIFORNIA*
*LBS. LOST 40*

* * * * * * * *

**IN 1997, I FINALLY FOLLOWED** the advice a dietitian had given me 10 years earlier after making a study of my food intake: "If you cut back on your bread, pasta, and potato intake, plus exercise a little, you won't have a problem." Acting on this advice, I lost 60 pounds within a few months and have maintained that weight loss ever since.

—*SYLVIA W. STODDARD*
*HOLLY HILL, FLORIDA*
*LBS. LOST 65*

# FOUR DIET DON'TS

- Do not eat anything that comes from a bag, box, container, or wrapper.
- Do not eat take-out or drive-through food. Eat only what comes from your kitchen.
- Do not eat what other people offer you or bring to work.
- Do not order lunch at work; bring your own food that you made at home.

—*JILL MARIE DAVIS*
*WEEHAWKEN, NEW JERSEY*
*LBS. LOST 20*

I TRIED THAT DIET WHERE you're not supposed to eat after 8 p.m., and it turned me into an insomniac because I was so hungry. I was up for six hours after I stopped eating, and that's just stupid. The guys who write those diet books don't know you and your life, so don't be stupid and take it as gospel.

—RYAN
CHAPEL HILL, NORTH CAROLINA
LBS. LOST 10

• • • • • • • •

## DIET DATA
According to a 2004 report, 22 percent of Americans are concerned about the amount of sugar in their diets.

IT ALL COMES DOWN TO CALORIES and not ingesting more energy from food than you expend in any given day. But counting calories is not everyone's idea of a happy existence, so researching low-calorie foods and changing your diet to incorporate them will inevitably lower your caloric intake.

—A.M.
BROOKLYN, NEW YORK
LBS. LOST 10

• • • • • • • •

LOW CARBS AND WALKING were most successful. It was the first time that I felt like I wasn't being punished by dieting. I could still eat so many of my favorite things, and there are so many low-carb dessert options. It didn't feel like a diet!

—DANA LEAR
LAWRENCEBURG, KENTUCKY
LBS. LOST 125

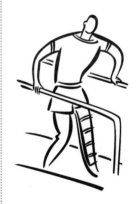

• • • • • • • •

PICK A DIET THAT'S REALISTIC. You can't tell yourself you're going to eat grapefruit for the rest of your life. Your body can't live on grapefruit. Jumping on a bandwagon isn't necessarily right for everyone.

—KATE CRONE
GREEN BAY, WISCONSIN

# WHAT THEY SAY ABOUT . . .

*They began as books: today the South Beach Diet and the Atkins Diet are worldwide systems, with interactive Web sites, packaged foods, and millions of followers. Some of our respondents shared their opinions of the pros and cons of each.*

**THE SOUTH BEACH DIET** is the only diet where I didn't feel hungry—after the first two weeks anyway. It was like someone flipped off a switch. Not being hungry was such a foreign feeling to me! I felt like my body was working the way it was supposed to.

> —*SANDI*
> *ALLENTOWN, PENNSYLVANIA*
> *LBS. LOST 60*

- - - - - - - - -

**I LOVE SOUTH BEACH** because it allows me to eat my favorite foods like berries, veggies, and even whole grains. The reason it works for me is because I got my husband to go on it, too, and I don't have to watch him eating bad things.

> —*SANDY URIBE*
> *SAN ANTONIO, TEXAS*
> *LOST TWO CLOTHING SIZES*

- - - - - - - - -

**MY MOST SUCCESSFUL EFFORT** was the South Beach Diet. But I think at the point where I started it almost anything would have worked because of my mental state: I was ready to change my habits, and it was about health. I did find that South Beach was more doable than Atkins, though, because it wasn't as restrictive. I think it's a healthy diet option.

> —*GEORGIA RAFF*
> *KIRKLAND, WASHINGTON*
> *LBS. LOST 55*

**MY HUSBAND AND I DID ATKINS.** It worked: I lost 40 pounds; he lost 55. Why did it work? Honestly? Because we love to drink, and you can keep drinking while you're on it. Well, you're not supposed to drink red wine, but white wine? Vodka? Gin? Bourbon? Yes. Kind of weird, considering you can't eat sugar, and most alcohol either has it, or is metabolized as fat.

—*ANONYMOUS*
*NORTHAMPTON, MASSACHUSETTS*
*LBS. LOST 40*

**ONE GIRL I KNOW WENT ON ATKINS** and took it as an excuse to raid Burger King every day (tossing aside the buns, of course).

—*J.A.*
*IOWA CITY, IOWA*

**I'VE TRIED THEM ALL, BUT ATKINS** was the only one that took off the weight for me. The diet works, but you have to stick with it. I was losing about five or eight pounds a week, and everyone could tell the difference. Then I went on a vacation to the Bahamas, went off the diet so I could have a good time, and I gained everything back within two weeks.

—*ABBY*
*CHICAGO, ILLINOIS*
*LBS. LOST 20*

# BOOK IT!

**I READ BILL PHILLIPS'S** *Body for Life* and stuck to that plan. Six days a week, I went to the gym and did cardio and weight training. On the seventh, I rested. Six days a week, I ate frequent, smaller meals, each of which contained a protein, starch or grain, and vegetable. On the seventh, I ate anything I wanted. This plan worked because I didn't view it as a diet, but as a lifestyle change.

—*E.C.*
NEW YORK, NEW YORK
LBS. LOST *20*

**I FOUND AN APPROACH THAT** I really like in the diet book *Curves*. Initially, the book helps you discover if you're calorie sensitive or carbohydrate sensitive and offers the best approach for each. Then, after you reach your goal weight, they have a maintenance routine that helps you to reset your metabolism to keep your weight from creeping back up. I found this to be very helpful.

—*JEAN NICK*
KINTNERSVILLE, PENNSYLVANIA
LBS. LOST *40*

**I READ DR. PHIL'S BOOK,** *Self Matters*, and realized a lot of my problem was that I wasn't willing to change my lifestyle to accommodate my health and well-being. I made the decision to commit to a workout routine, watch what I ate and make conscious decisions about what I was about to eat. I work out at Curves, and I started to notice the biggest change about six months into my diet and exercise plan. Although I was very frustrated that it did not happen overnight, I was determined to keep going, because eventually it would start to pay off. And it did! I've lost about 9 inches, 12 pounds, and a total of 8.2 percent of body fat.

—*K.K.*
KIRKLAND, WASHINGTON
LBS. LOST *12*

**I JUST FINISHED A BOOK ON HOW** to maintain a healthy lifestyle. These tips work for me: Never go on a diet, but never go off one either. You must constantly be aware without obsessing. Make simple adjustments to every day eating. Enjoy food in moderation and eat with the idea to empower your health.

—*LOUISE*
*NEW YORK, NEW YORK*

. . . . . . . . .

**I HAVE NOTHING AGAINST DIET BOOKS** except that you really never know which diets are going to work for you until you give them a shot. And if they don't work and you already bought the book, you're out of luck. And that's $20 you could have spent on ice cream.

—*SHIRL MAWHINNEY*
*PORTERSVILLE, PENNSYLVANIA*
*LBS. LOST 31*

**DO NOT SUBSCRIBE TO THE MYTH** that eating fat-free or sugar-free foods, counting points, or drinking shakes will solve an issue that took a couple of decades to do a number on you. Design a plan for yourself based on realistic goals and the time and resources you have to commit to the huge change you want to make. The slower you lose the weight, the longer you will keep it off. If you combine healthy eating, exercise, and strength-training, you will see and feel more of the benefits of your hard work.

—*JILL MARIE DAVIS*
*WEEHAWKEN, NEW JERSEY*
*LBS. LOST 20*

• • • • • • • •

**I HAVE BEEN ON SEVERAL DIETS,** but the most effective one was known as food combining. You can't mix meats and starches, but you can have plenty of one food group at one sitting. The first week called for nothing but fruit: I had been a meat-and-potatoes kind of guy, and eating nothing but fruit for a week was a real shock to my system. I quickly lost 25 pounds, and I have often gone back to it when I need to lose a few.

—*GORDON ALLISON*
*MARIETTA, GEORGIA*
*LBS. LOST 25*

• • • • • • • •

**I LET MYSELF EAT WHAT** I want on the weekends, I work out a couple of times a week, and during the week I eat mostly healthy food. I never keep junk food in my apartment. If I have a sweet tooth, I eat yogurt or I go to the store and buy a single serving of the junk food I'm craving. Whenever I want to eat something that's especially high in carbs, like pasta, I put a protein with it to make it more balanced.

—*J.H.*
*GLENDALE HEIGHTS, ILLINOIS*
*LBS. LOST 20*

**I eat small quantities all day long and keep moving. It seems like an efficient way to keep myself going without ever feeling overly hungry.**

—*JANE B.*
*GIBBSTOWN,*
*NEW JERSEY*
*LBS. LOST 15*

**RELAX! FIND TIME EACH DAY** to practice stress management to help regulate stress hormones, which can contribute to weight gain. It helps to turn off the TV and the Internet a few hours before bed. Doing simple stretching exercises or relaxing with yoga videos works, too.

—*KAT CARNEY*
*LOS ANGELES, CALIFORNIA*
*LBS. LOST* **90**

. . . . . . . .

" Tricking yourself by spicing up bland diet foods will keep you satisfied. Just make sure that whatever you add is "diet" or low in fat, so you don't end up gaining more weight! "

—*LISA DOUGLASS*
*SAN FRANCISCO, CALIFORNIA*

. . . . . . . .

**THE COMEDIAN HENNY YOUNGMAN** once told a joke that I think about every time I hear someone talking about the latest, greatest diet craze. He said, "My wife is on a diet where she only eats bananas and coconuts. She hasn't lost any weight, but boy can she climb a tree." I think that about sums up my feelings about these insane diets where you only eat grapefruit or you don't eat any bread. It's lunacy.

—*ANONYMOUS*
*ELLSWORTH, OHIO*
*LBS. LOST* **5**

# WHAT THEY SAY ABOUT. . .

*Various other commercial systems work for many dieters. Here's what they said about LA Weight Loss, Jenny Craig, and NutriSystem.*

**I THINK LA WEIGHT LOSS SAVED MY LIFE.** After I lost my weight, I noticed a mass in my left breast, so I had a mammogram and sonogram, and it turned out to be cancer.

> —KAREN BUFFUM
> ROUND ROCK, TEXAS
> LBS. LOST 25

• • • • • • • • •

**THERE WAS AN LA WEIGHT LOSS BRANCH** just 20 minutes from my home. It was easy to drop in for my one-on-one sessions three times a week; they usually only take five to ten minutes. I lost 72 pounds in just 37 weeks. It was one of the easiest things I've ever done in my life. The weight just came off. Now that I've lost the weight, I'm not the same person I was before: I'm a whole new me. I'm happier now than I ever was before.

> —DIANE SZYMANSKI
> SOUTH BEND, INDIANA
> LBS. LOST 72

• • • • • • • • •

**REGARDLESS OF THE DANGERS,** fad diets and programs like Jenny Craig that don't allow you to eat real food on your own schedule are far more likely to fail since it goes back to learning how to change. Anyone can lose weight following a strictly imposed regimen, but how will they do when they reach their goal and re-enter the real world of potlucks at work, buffets at parties, and buckets of movie popcorn?

> —ERICKA DUNHAM
> SEATTLE, WASHINGTON
> LBS. LOST 73

**A FEW MONTHS AGO,** I was checking into meal delivery services, figuring it would be great if someone else did the cooking and portioning. NutriSystem meals average out to about $3 each, and there are more than 100 meals from which to choose. The program is designed for you to eat three meals and two snacks a day, and you supplement the meals with fresh fruits and vegetables.

—KAT CARNEY
LOS ANGELES, CALIFORNIA
LBS. LOST 90

**I REALLY ENJOYED LA WEIGHT LOSS.** They teach you how to change your lifestyle. I learned how to cook differently and how to eat differently. The program has three parts: weight loss, stabilization, and maintenance. During the weight-loss phase, you go to one-on-one counseling three times a week. This worked well for me because you don't need a set appointment, you just drop in. They check your weight and blood pressure, suggest meal plans for you, and help guide your food choices.

—KAREN PHILLIPS
LANSING, ILLINOIS
LBS. LOST 42

**I'VE HAD SUCCESS WITH JENNY CRAIG.** Each week, I go there to weigh in, and they take my measurements once a month. I sit down with my counselor each week, and we talk about how the week went, what worked, what didn't, and what I can do better the next week.

—ANNMARIE PEARSON
GIG HARBOR, WASHINGTON
LBS. LOST 68

**DIET DATA**

Although four percent of Americans are currently on low-carb diets, only one in four of them is actually cutting a significant amount of carbs.

**THE ONLY WAY TO DIET** successfully is to know exactly what you are putting into your body. You have to know how many calories you are eating and whether they are bad or good. If you go on a diet for a limited time, you're just going to eat it back. You have to create a healthy eating lifestyle and stick to it.

—G.P.
IOWA CITY, IOWA

• • • • • • • • •

**FOR ME, IT'S ALL ABOUT PORTION SIZES.** I counted calories, read labels, and used online tools to figure out how many calories were in the foods I ate. In the beginning, I stayed under 1,600 calories a day, then lowered it to 1,500. If you make smart choices, that's a lot of food.

—AMANDA VEGA
SCOTTSDALE, ARIZONA
LBS. LOST 40

• • • • • • • • •

**I GAVE UP DAIRY AND CAFFEINE,** and my boobs have shrunk a whole size, which was a good thing for me. I'm not sure if it's because of the hormones in the dairy or what, but I'm pretty sure there's a connection.

—MARY
NEW YORK, NEW YORK
LBS. LOST 7

• • • • • • • • •

**IF YOU DENY YOURSELF,** you'll lose weight, but the minute you allow yourself that ice cream bar or that bag of chips, you'll be right back where you started, perhaps even heavier. It would be great if there were a magical cure to weight loss, a quick fix, but like anything in life, it takes hard work and focus. Eat well, get moving, and you'll see a difference.

—HOLLIE OVERTON

**MODIFY DIETS TO SUIT YOURSELF.** My husband suggested I try the Atkins diet. I thought it would be a good fit for me, except I didn't want to eat all of that high-fat food, such as eggs, sausage, and bacon. So I realized that you can follow the spirit of the diet but adjust it to avoid those high-fat foods. I ate more chicken and fish, but I still complied with the overall Atkins diet. It worked for me!

*—PAULINE T. MAYER
SMITHTOWN, NEW YORK
LBS. LOST 35*

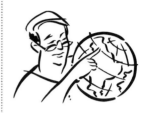

**MY DOCTOR RECENTLY PUT ME** on a kidney stone diet. (I'd been developing kidney stones for years.) He actually told me to drink so much water that it would be coming out my ears. When I told my granddaughter, who is 11, that I was on a kidney stone diet she asked me what kidney stones taste like. I told her I didn't know and I hope I never find out.

*—E.C.
WINONA, OHIO
LBS. LOST 5*

## THE DNA DIET

Using the new science of nutrigenomics, the Center for Health Enhancement in Santa Monica, California offers eating plans tailored to clients' genetic profiles.

**ONE SIMPLE CHANGE MADE** a big difference for me: I stopped eating carbohydrates after 5 p.m. Now my supper doesn't include any carbs, but I do still have them at breakfast and lunchtime.

*—LIZA
OREM, UTAH
LBS. LOST 17*

**THE CEREAL DIET IS A GOOD WAY** to lose weight in two weeks. It is just a bowl of cereal at breakfast and lunch and then a balanced supper. And you can eat unlimited fruits and vegetables all day.

*—JOSIE
NORTHANTS, ENGLAND
LBS. LOST 9*

# LOW THIS, LOW THAT

**LOW CARB:** The theory behind the diet sounds simple: If you restrict the amount of carbohydrates you consume, your body will begin to burn stored body fat as an energy source through a process called ketosis. Unfortunately, ketosis is an unhealthy condition to maintain for long, and one of the primary reasons most people fail on this type of diet long-term.

There are a number of popular fad diets today that advocate the low-carb, high-protein approach to weight loss. However, there is concern over the long-term effects due to the high level of animal proteins and total fats that these diets allow. Diets rich in animal fats are generally associated with heart disease and other health conditions.

**LOW FAT:** Low-fat diets became popular because they were meant to be not only good for losing weight, but also good for your overall health. Since one gram of fat contains twice as many calories as one gram of protein or carbohydrate, and calorie intake is a key factor in weight loss, a low-fat diet *should* lead to weight loss.

But many low-fat foods contain higher levels of sugar in order to replace flavor that is lost when the fat is removed. Lower-fat foods are often still calorie-laden.

**LOW CALORIE:** The low-calorie diet relies on the simple truth that if you burn more calories than you take in, you will lose weight. While it is true that calories are a key factor for healthy, sustainable weight loss, remember that a low-calorie eating plan may not necessarily be a healthy one, if it is filled with lower-calorie foods that are also empty-calorie foods that do not provide a lot of nutrients.

You will never feel full or satisfied on a low-calorie diet if those calories that you eat lack good nutrition. Remember to select foods that are high in nutritional value.

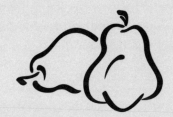

## DIET DATA

The best known diets in American are (in order of familiarity):

Atkins

Weight Watchers

Jenny Craig

SlimFast

Richard Simmons

Grapefruit Diet

Subway Diet

Metabolife

South Beach Diet

NutriSystem

**WRITE DOWN EVERYTHING** you eat in a notebook or diary. Make sure to include not just what you ate, but how much: one chicken breast, 15 tortilla chips, two cups of chili, etc. You'll find you'll avoid junk food and sweets—or at least limit the quantities you eat—if you know you'll be writing it down. Seeing what you've eaten in print can be pretty shocking if you're not eating right.

—*D.T.*
*Los Angeles, California*
*LBS. LOST 34*

• • • • • • • • •

**THE DIET ROLLER COASTER HAPPENS** because people think they can avoid changing their life by giving up cake for two weeks: it doesn't work that way. You have to find natural food that you like and really change your diet.

—*Fred*
*Washington, D.C.*
*LBS. LOST 17*

• • • • • • • • •

**DRINK LOTS OF WATER.** I'm 60 years old, and I've struggled with my weight since I was 38, particularly in my midsection. I drink 8 to 10 glasses of water a day. I make sure to always have water with me. For example, I bring a bottle in the car and refill it on breaks at work. Some of my coworkers have huge, 64-ounce water bottles. They can fill those bottles up once and sip all day.

—*Ruth*
*Orem, Utah*
*LBS. LOST 70*

# Sweet Temptation: Dealing with Your Favorite Sinful Snacks

*I f weight loss is the war, giving up your favorite indulgences is hand-to-hand combat. Here's how to identify your trigger foods, give them up if you have to, and work to control them if you can't.*

**WHAT ARE MY TRIGGER FOODS?** May I say everything? Let's just focus on chocolate, bread, and cheese. So if I stock my house only with what I should eat and plan simply prepared meals, I'm most successful.

—ALLAN JAFFE
   PETALUMA, CALIFORNIA

**COOKIES AND PIZZA ARE MY DOWNFALL! I COULD LIVE ON BOTH.**

—J.S.
IOWA CITY, IOWA
LBS. LOST 25

**I HAVE A STANDING ORDER WITH** a Belgian chocolate shop on Robson Street in Vancouver. Whenever I receive it in the mail every six months, guilt overcomes me as though I'm opening porn. I don't care that it puts on the pounds—OK, I do care—but I'll eat it anyway. Life's too fleeting not to give in to your aching passions every now and then.

—*EDGAR POMA*
*SAN FRANCISCO, CALIFORNIA*
*LBS. LOST 30*

* * * * * * * *

" I exercise willpower at the store; this way I don't have to be strong at home. I simply don't buy things like cookies, candy, and chips. "

—*DEANNA*
*MACUNGIE, PENNSYLVANIA*

* * * * * * * *

**I'M A TACO BELL FREAK;** that's how I put on my weight. When I got out of the Navy, I weighed 175 pounds. Then I met my girlfriend, and she worked at the mall, and I would pick her up. We would always stop to eat at Taco Bell. I was eating double-stuffed burritos at 10:30 p.m. A year later I was up to 195 pounds. Taco Bell is a guilty pleasure I'll probably never give up.

—*JOE*
*MILWAUKEE, WISCONSIN*
*LBS. LOST 25*

# YOU ARE HOW YOU EAT

One of the main reasons for overeating is not focusing on the actual act of eating. If you just grab one thing, shove it down, then grab the next, you never have time to think about what you're doing, to listen to your own body cues to see if you're really hungry. Also, you can't actually enjoy what you are putting into your mouth.

It's not what you eat; it's how you eat it.

—*ERIKA MALZBERG*
*SAN FRANCISCO, CALIFORNIA*
*LBS. LOST 20*

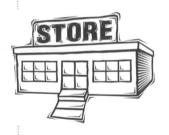

**IF I HAD A TASTE FOR SOME CHOCOLATE** at work I would not simply walk to the nearest vending machine and buy a Kit-Kat bar. I would walk down the seven flights of stairs and three blocks to the little store, and buy the candy there. Then I'd walk back up the stairs to my desk. At least I got some exercise in the process.

—*MICHELLE WATSON*
*CHURCHILL, OHIO*
*LBS. LOST 20*

**PASTA: I COME FROM AN ITALIAN FAMILY** where pasta and wine were on the table for just about every meal we had. And I guess old habits die hard. It's hard to give it up because it feels like my body really needs it. To make matters worse I like to top the pasta with parmesan cheese whenever it's available. And in my house it's always available.

—*RAY VINCET*
*LAVALE, MARYLAND*
*LBS. LOST 12*

# WHEN YOU GET A CRAVING . . .

**GO FOR A WALK.** You have to get yourself away from the things that you are craving, and unless it's twigs and berries, you won't find them outside on your walk.

> —*BRITTANY TALIAFERRO*
> *MEYERSDALE, PENNSYLVANIA*
> *LBS. LOST 7*

**I USE A COMBINATION OF WATER AND COMPUTER CHESS:** I realize this is a little out of the ordinary. First, drink as much water as you can stand. Then, you have to find something to occupy your mind. For me, the more I have to think about some other activity, the less I think about the food I want. So I get on my computer and challenge the chess program. There is no way you can think about chocolate cake when you're worried about the computer taking your queen.

> —*GEORGE ALLEN*
> *FROSTBURG, MARYLAND*
> *LBS. LOST 20*

**WHEN I WALK BY A BOX OF WARM,** delicious doughnuts in my office, I walk right up to the box and cut off just a sliver of a doughnut and relish the bite! I feel decadent, but not guilty, and if I get a sweet tooth in the afternoon, I can have a second sliver so as not to feel like I ate the whole box!

> —*SAMANTHA PHILLIPS*
> *ATLANTA, GEORGIA*
> *LBS. LOST 25*

**WHEN I HAVE A STRONG CRAVING** I tell myself that if I really want those Doritos a half hour from now, I'll have them. Nine times out of ten when the time is up I've been distracted by another activity or a healthier food.

> —*VERONICA LORSON FOWLER*
> *AMES, IOWA*
> *LBS. LOST 18*

**KEEP YOURSELF BUSY:** idle hands are the devil's workshop! You'll be surprised how quickly you lose interest in that food if you find yourself something productive to do. Clean your place, run the sweeper, clean out the fridge. . . well, you might not want to do *that*, come to think of it.

—TINIKA GILL
HYATTSVILLE, MARYLAND
LBS. LOST 10

• • • • • • • •

**WHEN I NEED A SUGAR FIX,** I reach for a handful of pretzels or a 100-calorie pack of Chips Ahoy cookies.

—STEPHANIE CONE
MONROE, IOWA
LBS. LOST 20

• • • • • • • •

**TO STOP A SUGAR CRAVING,** eat a pickle! No kidding, it really works.

—SANDI
ALLENTOWN, PENNSYLVANIA
LBS. LOST 60

• • • • • • • •

**I USUALLY GO TO BED** if the craving gets too bad. Once you fall asleep and wake up the next day, the cravings are usually gone—at least for a little while.

—BILL DAUGHERTY
FROSTBURG, MARYLAND
LBS. LOST 17

• • • • • • • •

**JUST GIVE IN.** If you are dying for Oreos and can think of nothing but Oreos, have one or two. That's better than letting the craving build to the point where you put away a box of them in one sitting.

—BRIAN HORZICH
WHEELING, WEST VIRGINIA
LBS. LOST 11

**MEDITATE.** I know it sounds crazy, but if you just find a quiet place where you can sit with your eyes closed, you can make the cravings stop. It's mind over matter and not as hard as you might think. Do it in the dark if you can. Just sit and close your eyes: Think of something else. You have to learn to concentrate on clearing your mind. If you sit like that for just 10 or 15 minutes, you will feel very refreshed.

> —*ERICA GRAHAM*
> *ACCIDENT, MARYLAND*
> *LBS. LOST 15*

**EAT SOMETHING ELSE.** Fill your stomach to make the rumblings stop, but you have to do it with something healthy. I don't think it's a good idea to try to ignore hunger pains; it just intensifies cravings. When I get hungry, I'm eating. You have to learn not to eat unless you are actually hungry. But at those times like late at night when I used to eat Doritos now I eat an apple.

> —*ANGELA*
> *FROSTBURG, MARYLAND*
> *LBS. LOST 11*

**IF THE CRAVING GETS TOO BAD,** offer yourself a reward for fighting it. Take yourself to the movies (no popcorn) or buy yourself something that you've had your eye on. Of course you don't want to make a habit of this, or you'll end up broke as well as fat.

> —*DONNA BURDON*
> *LAVALE, MARYLAND*
> *LBS. LOST 13*

**MANY OF MY FRIENDS WHO ARE NOW** in their mid-30s and starting to get some love handles like to think they can diet but still have their beer. It just doesn't work that way. If you are on a serious diet, you have to give up alcohol.

—*PHIL LYNCH*
*PITTSBURGH, PENNSYLVANIA*
LBS. LOST *15*

. . . . . . . .

" Here's a way to satisfy chocolate cravings: Chocolate soy milk. It has a really rich chocolate taste—even richer than regular chocolate milk. It has only about 150 calories in an eight-ounce glass. "

—*MARY*
*ALLENTOWN, PENNSYLVANIA*
LBS. LOST *25*

. . . . . . . .

**BREAD: I GREW UP IN A FAMILY** where there was some kind of bread on the table for every single meal. If we weren't eating white bread sandwiches for lunch, it was biscuits, rolls or buns with dinner. Those are tough habits to break. I almost feel like the meal's not complete without bread.

—*M.K.M.*
*OWINGS, MARYLAND*
LBS. LOST *5*

**YOU CAN'T BE A BEER DRINKER**—even a moderate one—and kid yourself that you are dieting. I have a friend who claims he can drink six light beers a day and still lose weight, as long as he works out. The only thing he's losing is more brain cells and a chance at getting in those 32"-waist jeans ever again.

—*STEVE O'HODNICK*
*SWISSVALE, PENNSYLVANIA*
*LBS. LOST 5*

• • • • • • • •

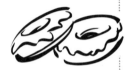

**DONUTS ARE MY DOWNFALL.** It's bread, sugar, and fat in the same item. I have a hard time saying no to them, so I don't keep that stuff in the house—although my husband buys and then hides them.

—*ANDREA COX*
*GRAND LAKE, COLORADO*
*LBS. LOST 30*

• • • • • • • •

**PEEPS: YOU KNOW,** those yellow marshmallow treats you see around Easter that are shaped like little chicks? I buy those in huge quantities and freeze them. I love them! The trick is to let them sit out and get a little stale: I know it sounds weird, but you have to try it. The good news is that they are low in fat. The bad news is, with as many as I eat, that's little comfort.

—*BERNICE ZLATOS*
*YOUNGSTOWN, OHIO*
*LBS. LOST 5*

• • • • • • • •

**FAST FOOD:** I just don't have the time or the money to eat right so it seems like every day I find myself at Burger King or McDonald's. It's just so cheap and easy. And they are constantly pounding on you with the advertising.

—*KADESH HARDIE*
*FROSTBURG, MARYLAND*
*LBS. LOST 8*

Forrest Gump said life is like a box of chocolates, but it's going to be a short life if you eat the whole box.

—*MARTIN SEABECK*
*FOMBELL,*
*PENNSYLVANIA*
*LBS. LOST 9*

I CANNOT MAKE IT THROUGH a day without dark chocolate. Denying myself does not work. But that's my only vice. In fact, if asked to choose between a glass of wine or a 70-percent-cocoa chocolate bar, I always choose the latter!

—L.G.
ATLANTA, GEORGIA
LBS. LOST 26

## DIET DATA

Americans spent $24 billion in 2003 on candy and ate 3 billion pounds of chocolate. In fact, we consumed nearly as much sugar as poultry.

CHOCOLATE IS MY WEAKNESS. To try to keep it under control, I buy chocolate only in those mini-bar sizes. Of course, it's hard to eat just one: I stash the bag in the high cabinet above my refrigerator so I have to make an effort to get to them. If my family sees me dragging a kitchen chair over to that cabinet, they know I'm searching for chocolate, and they can tease me accordingly.

—DAPHNE
OREM, UTAH
LBS. LOST 47

BEER: COME ON, WHO DOESN'T LIKE BEER? I just can't give it up. I tried light beer, but it's just like drinking water. If you're going to drink light beer, you might as well just drink Perrier.

—SANDRA FONKOUA
SILVER SPRING, MARYLAND
LBS. LOST 4

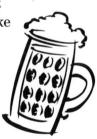

MY WORST CRAVINGS ARE FOR SALTY FOODS, like chips, and the worst time of day for me is mid-afternoon. The best way I've found to combat it is to drink water to fill me up. At work, I'll just walk to the water cooler, which is close to my desk. This helps me to resist the urge to go downstairs to the cafeteria to buy snacks.

—JENNIFER
READING, PENNSYLVANIA
LBS. LOST 70

**SUGARY CEREAL: I'M NOT PICKY,** I'll eat Froot Loops, Cap'n Crunch, Cocoa Pebbles. I love them all. I don't eat them just for breakfast, either, but for all three meals—sometimes in the same day. That can't be good.

—*JAMES SALTER*
*YOUNGSTOWN, OHIO*
*LBS. LOST 17*

• • • • • • • •

**ICE CREAM IS ONE OF THE BIGGEST** sins when dieting. I used to make ice cream milk shakes late at night because they hit the spot. Recently, I decided to make the switch to Healthy Choice low-fat ice cream and ice cream bars at night because they taste basically the same.

—*BUZZ ORR*
*EVANSTON, ILLINOIS*
*LBS. LOST 15*

• • • • • • • •

**ONCE I ATE A WHOLE BAG** of caramel-flavored rice cakes when I really just wanted a taste of my daughter's Cracker Jacks. You'll eat a lot less if you let yourself have the real thing—and enjoy it.

—*NATALIE GROSDAYK*
*JAMAICA ESTATES, NEW YORK*
*LBS. LOST 12*

• • • • • • • •

## SNACK FACT

Chocolate is the number one craved food in America.

**BAGELS WITH CREAM CHEESE:** I have to pass two bagel places on my way to work each day. Sometimes I can pass the first one without stopping, but I rarely make it past both of them without pulling in. I've had people tell me that eating the bagel without the cream cheese wouldn't be so bad. But to me that's like eating a pizza without the mozzarella cheese on top.

—*BRENT ALEXANDER*
*MIDLAND, MARYLAND*
*LBS. LOST 9*

**ONE STRATEGY THAT WORKS** for me is saving treats for a worthwhile event. For example, I'd rather have a good dessert in a nice restaurant than a handful of store-bought cookies.

—*STACY PHILLIPS*
*LOS ANGELES, CALIFORNIA*

＂**My mom told me you can't kid yourself that you're on a diet if you're eating Twinkies.** ＂

—*STEVEN A. PARSONS JR.*
*FT. ASHBY, WEST VIRGINIA*
*LBS. LOST 11*

**MAYONNAISE:** Once I started dieting I realized how much I use it. And when I read the label on the jar and saw how much fat was in there, it almost made me sick. I mean, I knew it was fattening, but I didn't know it was that fattening. Miracle Whip works pretty well as a substitute.

—*MARCY CHILDS*
*FROSTBURG, MARYLAND*
*LBS. LOST 7*

**MICROWAVE POPCORN:** Hardly a night goes by when my wife and I don't eat a big bowl of buttery popcorn. Sometimes I even make two. I have a hard time watching a movie without the popcorn bowl on my lap.

—*MERLE USHER*
*POLAND, OHIO*
*LBS. LOST 10*

**I allow myself to eat one of anything I crave. You can't get fat off one of anything; it's six that becomes a problem.**

—*S.H.*
*MINOT,*
*NORTH DAKOTA*
*LBS. LOST 20*

**I NEED TO KEEP HEALTHY SNACKS** around to keep me from binging on my favorite foods later! I now pack granola bars and keep them in my office drawer. I used to eat chocolate in the middle of the day, but now I can reach for something a little healthier.

—*STACY SILVER*
*TORONTO, ONTARIO, CANADA*

• • • • • • • •

**LICORICE, ESPECIALLY THE CHERRY FLAVOR:** I swear I'm addicted to that stuff. Any diet I go on is going to have to give me license to continue eating it. Otherwise it's just not going to work.

—*ANN MARIE BUSH*
*POLAND, OHIO*
*LBS. LOST 15*

• • • • • • • •

**THE KEY IS NOT DENYING YOURSELF.** When you feel like you should be standing in a Depression era soup line for yesterday's boiled turnips, that's the moment you begin to lose the weight-loss battle.

—*DANIEL COLLINS*
*COCKEYSVILLE, MARYLAND*
*LBS. LOST 56*

• • • • • • • •

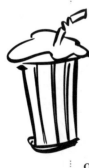

**ICE CREAM IS MY DOWNFALL:** I just love the creamy texture and especially the flavor Cookies 'n Cream. Now I buy the low-fat version or frozen yogurt. I open it up, scoop a small bite out with a teaspoon, close it back up, and put it in the freezer. I know that if I put some in a cup, I will be tempted to eat it all up and go back for more. This way, if I want another bite I have to walk to the freezer and take the time and energy to get the ice cream out again.

—*SAMANTHA PHILLIPS*
*ATLANTA, GEORGIA*
*LBS. LOST 25*

**PANCAKES, BUT NOT JUST PLAIN PANCAKES:** I have to eat them with as much butter and maple syrup as I can pile on. And I don't just eat them for breakfast. Pancakes can be eaten any time of the day or night. I love restaurants that serve breakfast food around the clock. I've spent many a late night guzzling down syrup and scooping up butter with my pancakes at those places.

—*BARRY FITTERER*
*CUMBERLAND, MARYLAND*
*LBS. LOST 11*

**No Krispy Kremes, under any circumstances.**

—*BETTY SMITH*
*PITTSBURGH,*
*PENNSYLVANIA*

**SALTY SNACKS ARE MY DOWNFALL:** Cheetos, pistachios, dry-roasted peanuts. If they are there, I eat them.

—*DAVID HUBBELL*
*KIRKLAND, WASHINGTON*
*LBS. LOST 50*

**IF I HAVE A CRAVING FOR SOMETHING,** such as chips, I ask myself how much I really want them. Am I really hungry or just bored? Why do I want them? Often, I can resist long enough that the craving passes. But if a craving lasts more than a day, I give in.

—*DEANNA*
*MACUNGIE, PENNSYLVANIA*

**IF YOU'RE SICK OF MORNING OATMEAL,** then go ahead and have a cupcake. But just understand that there is a price to pay. With me, cupcakes are my Achilles heel. I don't deny myself completely: I just remember that those calories have to be worked off.

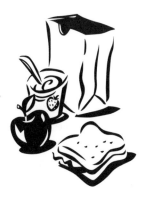

—*TIM LAKE*
*BADEN, PENNSYLVANIA*
*LBS. LOST 9*

**EVER HEARD OF PIRATE'S BOOTY?** It was touted as a healthy snack a couple years ago, and every grocery store was sold out of it. It's good stuff, but when they make healthy food that is too good, you eat the whole darn bag in one sitting.

—*ABBY*
*CHICAGO, ILLINOIS*
*LBS. LOST 20*

* * * * * * * *

" Rather than go cold turkey, eliminate one horrible thing from your diet each week. First week: sweets. Next week: beer. The week after: salt. You are allowed one little splurge, but don't make it a diet-ender and don't do it very often. "

—*STEPHEN MACKAY*
*SAN FRANCISCO, CALIFORNIA*
*LBS. LOST 10*

* * * * * * * *

**FRENCH FRIES:** I love them. I make them at home (baked) and count out a certain amount. That is the hardest part. Another trigger food is French bread; now I get multigrain baguette bread.

—*LEESA*
*REDMOND, WASHINGTON*
*LBS. LOST 27*

**IF YOU ARE DIETING OR TRYING** to eat healthier and you don't allow yourself a few indulgences here and there, what is the point? I have always believed that life is too short to have to worry about what I'm eating and how many calories it is. I want to eat what I want when I want to eat it. So, if you just can't get rid of that craving, eat some ice cream, but in a small portion. And if you can't control it at all, then drink water; water is the true key.

—*STEPHANIE CONE*
   *MONROE, IOWA*
   *LBS. LOST 20*

• • • • • • • •

**CAKES, COOKIES, AND ICE CREAM** top the list: I can't get enough of them. My girlfriend wants to kill me because every time I go to the grocery store, I come back with one of those pre-made cookie dough packages and manage to throw them in the oven and eat all but a few, which I share with her. There's no way to control your cravings, but living with someone who yells at you for eating badly is the only way I can cut down.

—*A. ORR*
   *CHICAGO, ILLINOIS*
   *LBS. LOST 10*

• • • • • • • •

**MY GREATEST DIETING DOWNFALL** is carbohydrates, mostly in the form of any kind of potato or pasta. I do have cravings for these things and have learned to control my portions. I try not to have two carbs together during one meal. I resist pasta and potatoes by reaching for fruits or sugar-free Popsicles. I do, at times, give in, but the guilt is definitely not worth it.

—*ANONYMOUS*
   *BIRMINGHAM, ALABAMA*
   *LBS. LOST 30*

## SNACK FACT

The top desserts—fruit, ice cream, cookies, and cake— make up two-thirds of all desserts served in America.

**IT'S MUCH BETTER TO JUST EAT WHAT** you want when a craving hits. As long as you don't have ten candy bars, you'll be fine. I used to try to substitute all of the healthy things, like carrots and air-popped popcorn, but all that happened is that I got stuffed. My cravings didn't go away. So I'd also eat the candy bar, piling on even more calories and fat. But I was too full to enjoy it, plus I felt guilty.

—*P.O.*
*NEW BRUNSWICK, NEW JERSEY*
*LBS. LOST 50*

* * * * * * * *

" Do not keep any junk food in your house. You're not going to drive somewhere to get it. "

—*COLLEEN WOZNIAK*
*AURORA, ILLINOIS*
*LBS. LOST 60*

* * * * * * * *

**I BUY THOSE LITTLE POUCHES OF FRUIT** snacks for my kids to put in their lunches for school, but then I sit there and munch on them all day long. They just taste so darn good! I tried telling myself that maybe they were actually healthy because they have the word "fruit" in them, but then I read the label. It's the same as thinking you are getting your daily share of dairy by eating cheesecake because it has the word "cheese" in it.

—*FELIX DELERME*
*GREENFORD, OHIO*
*LBS. LOST 5*

**JIF CREAMY PEANUT BUTTER:** I eat that for lunch almost every day. It is heavy on the fat. My mom says I've been eating that since I could eat solid foods. I don't plan to stop anytime soon.

—PATRICK CALIENDO
POLAND, OHIO
LBS. LOST 13

• • • • • • • •

**ONE OF THE BEST THINGS** I've found to combat a chocolate craving is chocolate pudding. Another thing that helps a sweet tooth is to take vanilla yogurt, or even fruit-flavored yogurt, and freeze it. It tastes like ice cream, but it's not sugary like frozen yogurt. It also has a bit of a tangy taste, which I like.

—SANDI
ALLENTOWN, PENNSYLVANIA
LBS. LOST 60

• • • • • • • •

**IT NEVER FAILS:** Every day at 3 p.m., I get a craving for something sweet. Instead of walking to the closest candy dish in my office, I have a couple of pieces of dried fruit. It completely ends the craving, and it is totally healthy.

—SAMANTHA PHILLIPS
ATLANTA, GEORGIA
LBS. LOST 25

• • • • • • • •

**I DON'T HAVE A SPECIFIC TRIGGER FOOD.** I love *all* food! I deal with this by allowing myself to eat whatever I want on Sundays. I will sit on the couch all day Sunday and eat, usually not very healthily. But if I let my body have its fill one day out of the week, I find that I can handle the cravings and wants a lot easier than if I denied myself.

—K.K.
KIRKLAND, WASHINGTON
LBS. LOST 12

My trigger food? Lay's Potato Chips, because I can't eat just one: one bag, that is.

—TERRY O'DONNELL
CANFIELD, OHIO
LBS. LOST 15

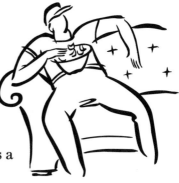

## DIET DATA

Americans today consume several hundred more calories per day than their predecessors did in the 1950s.

**I TOTALLY LOVE ICE CREAM** and could easily eat a whole pint two times a day. Luckily, there are some great low-carb ice creams on the market, and I usually make sure that I scoop the ice cream into a bowl and don't just sit down with a spoon and the carton, vowing to only eat a little bit and save the rest for later.

—Dana Lear
Lawrenceburg, Kentucky
LBS. LOST 125

• • • • • • • •

**KEEP SAFE INDULGENCES IN THE HOUSE;** for me, that's dark chocolate chips. When a craving hits, I grab a handful of chips and eat them one at a time. I find that the more you deprive yourself of foods that you love, the more obsessed with them you become.

—Mary Bright
Allentown, Pennsylvania

• • • • • • • •

**I TRY TO REWARD MYSELF WITH FOODS** that I really go crazy over, like Häagen Dazs's Bananas Foster ice cream. I treat myself to my favorite foods that I just can't give up when I accomplish a goal, whether it be work- or workout-related. The trick is to not make everything a special occasion. For example, "I woke up early this morning: This deserves a bowl of ice cream!"

—Q.S.
New York, New York

• • • • • • • •

**I MAKE STOVE TOP STUFFING** as a side dish with just about every meal. I'm totally hooked. I wonder if there is a detox center for stuffing addicts?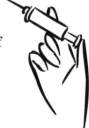

—F.W.
Poland, Ohio
LBS. LOST 10

**FOR HEALTH REASONS,** I was forced to stop eating many things I loved a few years back. No more bacon, no more gravy, no more biscuits for breakfast. It was like losing old friends.

—*FELIX*
*CHAPEL HILL, NORTH CAROLINA*
*LBS. LOST 25*

**DON'T BE SEDUCED BY THE SALES** at the grocery store or bullied by your children. You can't eat what you don't buy; make your list and stick to it.

—*SHELLEY GLADSTONE*
*ATLANTA, GEORGIA*
*LBS. LOST 15*

**MY HUSBAND WAS JUMPING** on me about eating too many M&Ms, so I told him I would only eat the green ones. If I have learned anything as a mother, it is that green foods are good for you.

—*CHRISTINA QUATCHAK*
*UNITY, OHIO*
*LBS. LOST 10*

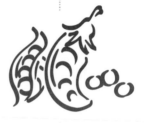

**TO RESIST THIS CRUELLY PLOTTED** array of Twinkies, Ding-Dongs, and Choco-Diles, I look at the hideous, bloated mascots that adorn such packaging. When I stare into the cold gaze of Twinkie the Kid, for example, I understand fully that his goal is for us all to look just like him—a rotund, misshapen mass with disturbingly high levels of fructose and hydrogenated vegetable oils. Is it any coincidence that the man wields a lasso? Each time I peer into a vending machine, the abject terror it brings usually convinces me to go for the low-fat trail mix instead.

—*J.A.*
*IOWA CITY, IOWA*
*LBS. LOST 15*

Brush your teeth and your craving will likely pass. And I'm not just saying that because I'm a dentist. . .

—*ANONYMOUS*
*TORONTO, ONTARIO, CANADA*
*LBS. LOST 12*

**WHENEVER I WANT CHOCOLATE** (which is pretty much any time my eyes are open), I remind myself of all the trouble those kids got into in *Willie Wonka and the Chocolate Factory.* That movie does a good job of showing how evil chocolate is and how it can ruin you. Get a craving and put that movie in the VCR. It will be cured immediately. Nobody wants to blow up like a balloon or get shrunk to the size of a thimble.

—*D.H.*
*LEETONIA, OHIO*
*LBS. LOST 13*

• • • • • • • •

**IF I DON'T EAT SUGAR FOR A FEW DAYS**, I don't crave it any more. What you crave is often what your body is addicted to!

—*DEEDEE MELMET*
*SONOMA, CALIFORNIA*
*LBS. LOST 50*

• • • • • • • •

**I KEEP SOME HERSHEY'S KISSES** at hand all the time. I even have some in my desk at work. If I need chocolate I allow myself one and only one. Maybe two.

—*CINDY KROEPIL*
*CHURCHILL, OHIO*
*LBS. LOST 10*

The foods that are the toughest for me to ignore are generally made of chocolate. Heck, I'd probably eat chocolate-covered cotton.

—*DANIEL COLLINS*
*COCKEYSVILLE, MARYLAND*
*LBS. LOST 56*

# Taste Test: Tips on Healthy Eating

Experts say the key to losing weight is to burn off more calories than you take in. But if it's really so simple, why is dieting so hard? (And we wonder just how many of those experts are still on diets, too!) Here are tips from weight-loss winners about eating better, which might make the fight just a little bit easier.

**TRY TO ENVISION YOUR BODY** as a vehicle and food as a fuel source. Your body will be at its maximum performance if you fill it with premium as opposed to unleaded.

—BETHANY AMBROSE
BETHESDA, MARYLAND
LBS. LOST 5

**STOP DRINKING COFFEE.**

—PAULINE T. MAYER
SMITHTOWN,
NEW YORK
LBS. LOST 35

**I USED TO PUT SALT ON MY SALT,** you might say. Then I switched to that imitation salt and now hardly ever use any of that either, which is another benefit of changing your diet. It helped me get my taste buds back.

—*DANIEL COLLINS*
*COCKEYSVILLE, MARYLAND*
LBS. LOST *56*

• • • • • • • •

**"A blender is a girl's best friend. I don't have time to eat breakfast so I whip up a fruit smoothie almost every morning—frozen fruit, bananas to make it creamy, nonfat yogurt and milk. Even my kids like them. "**

—*JESSICA ROTHMAN*
*NEW YORK, NEW YORK*
LBS. LOST *25*

• • • • • • • •

**INSTEAD OF A MEAL OF 2 1/4 CUPS** of pasta at about 450 calories, have a cup of pasta mixed with a cup of steamed vegetables and a cup of steamed sliced mushrooms. Total calories equals 220. It's colorful, filling, and good for you!

—*SUSIE GALVEZ*
*RICHMOND, VIRGINIA*
LBS. LOST *121*

**HEALTHY FOOD CAN BE THE BEST** tasting food there is; it's that fake diet stuff that's so depressing. I try to find pleasure in the things I can still eat. I grow vegetables so I know they will be the best vegetables ever, I bake bread. I still eat very well in terms of flavor. You can't beat a fresh tomato from the garden, but try feeding me a low-calorie snack bar, and I'll cry.

—*FELIX*
*CHAPEL HILL, NORTH CAROLINA*
*LBS. LOST 25*

• • • • • • • •

**MY FAVORITE TIME TO EAT** is always first thing in the morning. For one it's the time of the day that I am usually the hungriest after sleeping all night. I think you enjoy food more when you really need it. And also I get up for work very early while the house is still quiet and everyone else is in bed. I've found that I can really enjoy eating more without all the craziness that usually exists in the house.

—*PAT BUFORD*
*BOARDMAN, OHIO*
*LBS. LOST 15*

• • • • • • • •

**I READ LABELS CONSTANTLY** and don't buy anything that contains more than ten grams of sugar. Because getting enough protein is an issue, I also try to buy products that are high in protein. I use protein bars, high protein cereals, Trader Joe's nonfat cottage cheese, cheeses, and fish. Gala apples, nectarines, and grapes have been my salvation. I have also found a wonderful substitute for Starbucks: Just buy flavored coffee beans at the grocery store and add Splenda and a creamer. It is delicious!

—*ANN MOUSNER*
*MURIETTA, CALIFORNIA*
*LBS. LOST 118*

## SLIM STAT

Heart disease ranks as the number one cause of death in men. Two ways to help prevent it: Maintain a healthy weight, and eat a diet rich in fruits, veggies and low-fat foods.

## FOOD FACT

Food advertisements promote mostly foods high in calories, fat, or sugar. Only two percent of food advertising is for fruits, vegetables, grains, and beans.

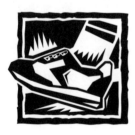

**I WOULD LOVE TO DO THE LEISURELY,** French, two-hour lunch thing, but get real; I'm lucky if I get 20 minutes to stuff something into my mouth. I recently started packing healthy "mini-meals" for work. Instead of my usual afternoon Starbucks run, I'll have a turkey sandwich on whole wheat, cheese sticks and fruit, or some yogurt. I find that having just a little bit of protein is a great pick-me-up for the afternoon fizzle.

—*NATALIE GROSDAYK*
*JAMAICA ESTATES, NEW YORK*
*LBS. LOST 12*

• • • • • • • •

**I USED TO HATE FRUIT,** but now fruit is an inexpensive, sweet fix for me. A banana and a cup of milk is a safe and healthy snack.

—*KARA*
*CHICAGO, ILLINOIS*
*LBS. LOST 217*

• • • • • • • •

**I ENJOY WHATEVER I EAT RIGHT AFTER** a workout, even if it's just celery sticks or a bran muffin. I think food tastes better after you get your blood pumping. I don't know if that's a mental thing or a physical thing, but it is almost always the case.

—*TERRY HARRINGTON*
*CUMBERLAND, MARYLAND*
*LBS. LOST 13*

• • • • • • • •

**I'M ALWAYS HAPPIEST EATING** stuff from my garden that I've grown myself with my own two hands. Nothing tastes better than tomatoes or potatoes or beans that I've tended to myself. Stuff from your garden is always healthy. I've never seen a garden with sticky buns growing in it. But if you ever do, please let me know.

—*WALT BULLOCK*
*BARRELVILLE, MARYLAND*
*LBS. LOST 9*

# THE SKINNY ON FATS

There is a sad truth about fat and weight loss: Your fat cells could not care less what type of fat you eat! Most of us are trying to eat the "good" fats or the "heart-healthy," monounsaturated fats (found in olive oil, peanut oil, canola oil, nuts, avocados, etc.) and polyunsaturated fats (found in sunflower oil, safflower oil, corn oil, soybean oil, sunflower seeds, etc.), since these two types of fat are less apt to form plaque on artery walls. While they are less likely to clog arteries leading to the heart, with respect to weight loss, you *can* eat too many of them. You can't pour olive oil all over your salad just because it's heart-healthy: Your fat cells love to store olive oil!

There are other types of fats. Cholesterol comes only from animal products; saturated fats are found in animal products, and in solid shortenings, egg yolks, lard, butter, margarine, cream, milk chocolate, and cocoa butter. Hydrogenated and partially hydrogenated fats are also known as "trans" fats. Trans fats are formed when hydrogen and pressure are added to liquid oils in order to form a more solid substance, such as Crisco shortening or margarine. Trans fats are generally hidden in processed foods or in baked goods such as muffins, cakes, pies, cookies, potato chips, and candy.

Trans fats pose perhaps a greater health risk than saturated fats. While saturated fats raise your LDL ("lousy," or bad, cholesterol), trans fats may do even more damage by not only raising your LDL, but actually lowering your HDL ("helpful," or good, cholesterol) at the same time.

Health-conscious consumers should read ingredient labels and watch out for shortening, hydrogenated or partially hydrogenated oil. The closer to the top of the ingredient list these oils appear, the more trans fat is contained in the product.

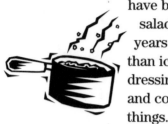

**My mother was a very British cook,** so everything was potatoes and vegetables boiled beyond recognition, plus fatty meats and sausages. I must have been in my fifties before I really discovered salad, and it's only been in the last couple of years that I've realized that salad can be more than iceberg lettuce smothered in blue cheese dressing. I try to eat things that are appealing and colorful, and I try to get flavor from natural things.

—*G.H.*
*CHAPEL HILL, NORTH CAROLINA*
*LBS. LOST 15*

. . . . . . . .

" Many soup, casserole, and sauce recipes call for cream. Instead, use fat-free evaporated milk. It adds rich flavor and zero fat. "

—*SUSIE GALVEZ*
*RICHMOND, VIRGINIA*
*LBS. LOST 121*

. . . . . . . .

**Try to eat more fresh foods.** I think of the French, who eat richer foods than we do, but are usually much thinner. One of the things that they do is eat much more fresh food. America is more of a packaged-food society. Fresh food tastes so much better, and it's better for you, too.

—*STACY PHILLIPS*
*LOS ANGELES, CALIFORNIA*

**I USED TO THINK** I was being good by skipping meals, especially breakfast. After all, why eat if you're not hungry? And sometimes I would be so busy that lunch was whatever floated by—fast food, a small salad, or even vending machine snacks. By the time I'd get home, I wouldn't just be hungry, I'd be ready to eat the entire refrigerator (doors included). I'd eat everything not bolted down. After some nutritional consultation, I learned that to lose weight I need to eat more (or at least more frequently). Now I don't let more than two or three hours go by without some food, preferably a little protein and carbs. I can't believe how much better I feel.

—*LHASA MANOR*
*PHILADELPHIA, PENNSYLVANIA*
*LBS. LOST 45*

• • • • • • • • •

**BE PREPARED FOR WHEN HUNGER STRIKES.** At my office, meetings start at 10 a.m., which is when I like to eat a mid-morning snack. So I take a box of raisins and a bottle of water into the meeting. No one seems to care if I snack on them. By controlling my hunger, I'm not ravenous by the time the meeting is over.

—*JEANNIE LOFRANCO*
*SAN JOSE, CALIFORNIA*
*LBS. LOST 99*

Get a really good sharp knife and learn how to use it (on your fruits and veggies, that is).

—*MAYTAL YARON*
*LOS ANGELES,*
*CALIFORNIA*
*LBS. LOST 15*

# FRUIT OF THE MONTH

The National Cancer Institute offers these uncommon fruits to incorporate into your diet:

**January:** dried fruit          **July:** nectarine
**February:** star fruit          **August:** cactus fruit
**March:** tamarillo              **September:** fig
**April:** Asian pear             **October:** persimmon
**May:** lime                     **November:** plantain
**June:** pluot                   **December:** kumquat

# OOHHMMMM ... GOOD!

When I was in school for nutrition, one of the teachers talked about this concept called Meditation on a Raisin. The basic idea was that if you put one raisin in your mouth and concentrated on that, and really thought about all the flavors, there wasn't that much difference between eating that one and eating a whole handful. Being healthy is a lot about slowing down, thinking about what you're eating, and really understanding what it is to be full or hungry.

—JASON T.
CHAPEL HILL, NORTH CAROLINA
LBS. LOST 20

Being a vegetarian is a great way to stay fit, slim, healthy, and at one with the world around you.

—BLAIRE BERGMAN

**LEARN THE ART OF CREATIVE SUBSTITUTION:** Prepare the foods you love with healthy ingredients to retain all the taste and satisfaction while reducing the calories and fat. The possibilities are endless once you get the hang of it.

—LOURDES FIGUEROA
MIAMI, FLORIDA
LBS. LOST 70

• • • • • • • •

**I ACTUALLY FIND THAT** I enjoy food better when someone else has prepared it. Food always seems to taste better when you eat at a restaurant or when your mom or a friend makes it. I think it's because when you go through the creation process yourself you subconsciously hold it against the food that you had to exert all that energy. You are much happier with the food when the only effort you have to make is getting it into your mouth.

—J.M.
BOARDMAN, OHIO
LBS. LOST 13

YOU DON'T HAVE TO TURN INTO one of these freaky label-readers who clog up the aisles in the supermarkets reading the ingredients of every item. But at least look at the total fat grams. For instance, take a look at the fat content of one of those little pre-packaged apple pies. Your eyes will pop out of your head. You'd be better off eating a couple of sticks of butter.

—CHUCK MANION
PITTSBURGH, PENNSYLVANIA
LBS. LOST 7

• • • • • • • • •

I MAKE A LOT OF SHAKES IN THE BLENDER, such as vanilla-flavored soy, high-fiber protein powder, crushed ice, and a few shakes of pumpkin pie spice. It's like eggnog.

—KATIE
OREM, UTAH
LBS. LOST 45

• • • • • • • • •

I HAVE A RULE THAT if I didn't bring it into work, I can't eat it. This keeps me away from the temptations in the cafeteria and snack bars. Instead I bring healthy snacks to work, such as fruit.

—JEANNIE LOFRANCO
SAN JOSE, CALIFORNIA
LBS. LOST 99

For a quick snack, I carry a Luna bar with me at all times.

—AMANDA VEGA
SCOTTSDALE, ARIZONA
LBS. LOST 40

# VEGGIE OF THE MONTH

The National Cancer Institute offers these uncommon vegetables to incorporate into your diet:

| | |
|---|---|
| **January:** tuber | **July:** garlic |
| **February:** calabaza squash | **August:** fennel |
| **March:** leek | **September:** chili pepper |
| **April:** tomatillo | **October:** ginger root |
| **May:** sprouts | **November:** greens |
| **June:** okra | **December:** parsnips |

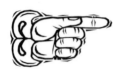

**EAT MORE FISH, CHICKEN, LEGUMES,** and nuts than red meat or the other white meat. Try to avoid eating the white stuff in general—bread, white rice, white pasta, and potatoes. Eat whole grains instead.

—*ALLAN JAFFE*
*PETALUMA, CALIFORNIA*

. . . . . . . .

" Read the labels on diet food. Many of those items are low in fat but are high in calories, salt, and carbohydrates. In the end, that's just as bad. You think you are being good but you're not losing weight because of bad food choices. "

—*RICHARD KAZIMER*
*NEGLEY, OHIO*
*LBS. LOST 22*

. . . . . . . .

**SOME THINGS THAT ARE HIGH** in protein are also high in fat—peanut butter, for instance. But I have found that the extra energy you get from protein is worth the extra fat.

—*DAN SANTOS*
*GREEN TREE, PENNSYLVANIA*
*LBS. LOST 21*

# MAKING THE MOST OF YOUR METABOLISM

Your metabolism is the process by which your body converts food into usable energy. A lot of important variables affect your metabolism. Any one of these factors or a combination of factors can greatly influence how your body utilizes its fuel and, more important, your ultimate weight-loss success. You and your spouse may eat the same meal, in the same quantity, but will burn the calories in that meal differently, based on your metabolic profiles.

Many factors play a role in determining how quickly you burn calories. A huge influence is genetics. If most of your blood relatives struggle with weight, the chances will be greater that you, too, will struggle.

Another factor to consider is your own personal "set-point," a weight that Mother Nature has somewhat pre-determined she would like you to weigh. Every attribute about you is written in your DNA. You may want to weigh 125 pounds, but if your DNA has predetermined that you weigh more, then no matter how hard you diet, you may not reach your goal of 125 pounds; and if you do reach it, you may not be able to maintain it for long. Generally, your set-point is the weight you reached in your mid-20s, or the weight that you always seem to come back to.

Another factor that may influence your metabolic rate is your body composition. Your current weight is derived partly from fat and partly from muscle. Muscle is more metabolically active: it can burn about 40-50 calories per pound per day, while fat may burn 2-3 calories per pound. Therefore, the person with more muscle may have a metabolic rate higher than a person with the same weight but a higher percentage of body fat.

**I TOOK PART IN A WEIGHT-LOSS STUDY.** They gave us meal plans and recipes to try and encouraged us to reduce our calories. The study was about people losing weight along with their dogs. The dogs made dietary changes, too, switching to low-fat dog food. The dietary changes they suggested worked for my dog, Spats, as well: he lost 13 pounds.

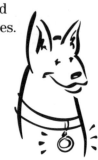

—*ROSEANN LOCASCIO*
*CHICAGO, ILLINOIS*
*LBS. LOST 30*

**Eat tons of popcorn, but skip the butter and salt. It's a very tasty snack and doesn't cost you hardly any calories.**

—*BRANDON BUCKLEY*
*YOUNGSTOWN, PENNSYLVANIA*
*LBS. LOST 3*

**VARIETY IS THE SPICE OF LIFE,** and it's also the most important thing to remember with a diet. You shouldn't get stuck eating just vegetables or just protein. Eat a little bit of everything, including sugars, but don't overdo it. When I started my diet, I tried to avoid milk products at all costs because of the high fat. But it just made me crave cheese all the more. I've found if I allow myself a little bit of it I don't think about it as often. And a little bit of anything isn't going to hurt.

—*MITZI SNYDER*
*ZELIENOPLE, PENNSYLVANIA*
*LBS. LOST 15*

**LOOK AT THE EUROPEANS.** I lived in London several years ago. Their eating habits are so different than ours. They enjoyed their biggest meal at lunch, and they have a sweet after every meal. But what I think was most important is that their portions are so much smaller than ours. I remember the family often would share a small chicken. In the United States, that would feed only two people!

—*STACY PHILLIPS*
*LOS ANGELES, CALIFORNIA*

**TWO OF THE MOST VALUABLE THINGS** I learned are to look for fiber in foods and to eat every couple of hours. I used to feel guilty about eating more than three meals a day. My concern was that people would think, "Look at that fat person who is always eating." But now I know it works to control my hunger and ultimately I eat less overall.

—*JEANNIE LOFRANCO*
*SAN JOSE, CALIFORNIA*
*LBS. LOST 99*

. . . . . . . .

**CUT IN HALF THE AMOUNT OF BUTTER** or oil called for in boxed side dishes such as rice, macaroni, potatoes, or other starchy foods. Instead add extra onions, carrots, celery, or other vegetables, and don't forget those spices. The dish will be tasty and satisfying without the extra fat.

—*SUSIE GALVEZ*
*RICHMOND, VIRGINIA*
*LBS. LOST 121*

. . . . . . . .

**LEARN HOW TO READ LABELS AND LEARN** which ingredients are OK to eat. Just because a product says it's low in carbs doesn't mean it doesn't contain enriched white flour, hydrogenated oils (trans fats), or high fructose corn syrup.

—*LINDA LANGDON*
*VANCOUVER, BRITISH COLUMBIA, CANADA*
*LBS. LOST MORE THAN 100*

. . . . . . . .

**WATCH YOUR SALAD DRESSING!** I know that sounds silly, but I've learned that the "healthy" salad with the wrong salad dressing can be have more fat than a cheeseburger. Check the nutritional contents on the dressing before you pat yourself on the back for eating healthy.

—*M.L.*
*PHILADELPHIA, PENNSYLVANIA*
*LBS. LOST 20*

**The best part of eating is the preparation. It's like foreplay before sex. The actual act is always somewhat of a letdown. The eating, I mean, not the sex.**

—*ANONYMOUS*
*STRUTHERS, OHIO*
*LBS. LOST 9*

# CALORIES: THEY'RE NOT ALL CREATED EQUAL

Like gasoline to a car or batteries to a flashlight, calories are the way your body gets fuel or power. There are however, different types of calories, depending on their source.

Carbohydrates are the body's primary energy source. They break down to glucose, or blood sugar, which your brain and central nervous system depend on for energy. Our muscles are fueled from the energy in carbs, but not all carbohydrates are the same. Fruits and vegetables, the healthiest of all carbohydrates, contribute the fewest total calories of any food. They are filled with antioxidants and phytochemicals, substances that help to protect against heart disease and cancer. The more colorful the fruit or vegetable, the greater the health benefits.

The protein calorie helps maintain, or repair, the body. It helps produce hormones, red blood cells, and antibodies for your immune system. Protein is found in chicken, turkey, fish, red meats, lamb, veal, pork, cheese, milk, yogurt, and to lesser degrees in nuts, and legumes. Most Americans eat two to three times the protein they actually need; the excess turns to body fat, of course.

The fat calorie is found everywhere. It truly does not matter what type of fat it is; the fat cells of your body are more than eager to store the fat calorie if you have consumed more than your body needs.

**THERE ARE SO MANY THINGS** we eat that contain eggs in one form or another, from breads to sweet little nothings, from sauces to salads. Sometimes the eggs are so concealed we don't even realize we are eating them. Keep in mind that the average egg yolk contains over two-thirds the recommended daily allowance of cholesterol. I have found that using egg substitutes works just as well.

—*VALERIE SHUSTECK*
*YOUNGSTOWN, PENNSYLVANIA*
*LBS. LOST 9*

• • • • • • • •

" Thinking of food as fuel for your body makes it a lot easier to choose nutritious, high-energy foods over empty-calorie junk foods. "

—*C. HUTCHINS*
*BARLING, ARKANSAS*

• • • • • • • •

**I MARRIED A WONDERFUL WOMAN,** but she has no interest in cooking. I am not an avid cook either, so the first year of marriage we mostly ate fruit, yogurt, cereal, raw vegetables, and sandwiches with the occasional pizza. This was quite a change from my mother's elaborate, home-cooked meals. Needless to say, I lost 20 pounds our first year of marriage!

—*BRIAN LEONARD*
*ENID, OKLAHOMA*
*LBS. LOST 20*

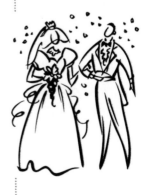

**FIND A COUPLE OF SNACK FOODS** that are good for you (or at least not bad for you) and make sure you always have them on hand at home and at work. For me, raw carrots are something I've always enjoyed, so I've made those my primary snack food. Another thing I enjoy are those jars of mixed pickled vegetables (they often have some combination of carrots, cocktail onions, pickles, cauliflower, baby carrots, and peppers in them).

—*D.T.*
*LOS ANGELES, CALIFORNIA*
*LBS. LOST 34*

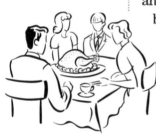

**BEFORE, I'D SERVE A ROAST WITH POTATOES,** rolls, and canned vegetables for supper. Now, I limit beef to three times a week and eat more chicken, turkey, and lean pork. I buy fresh vegetables, like broccoli, cauliflower, and green beans, and steam them in about a half inch of water in a saucepan, for about 20 minutes, until they're crisp-tender.

—*DIANE SZYMANSKI*
*SOUTH BEND, INDIANA*
*LBS. LOST 72*

**FOOD FACT**

Less than a quarter of Americans eat the recommended five fruits and vegetables a day.

**I LIVE IN THE SOUTH,** and you know how we eat everything: fried. So probably the hardest change for me was giving up fried foods. I started grilling, baking, broiling, boiling, steaming—everything *but* frying! And I learned after a while that I really began to taste my food, not the grease and the breading. I discovered that food was actually good! I also gave up southern-style sweet tea—I am a tea-aholic. It would be nothing for me to sit down and drink pretty close to a gallon of tea a night.

—*KANDI KIZZIAH*
*ROCKY MOUNT, NORTH CAROLINA*
*LBS. LOST 158*

**I EAT HEALTHY PROTEIN** (chicken and fish, not cheese and bacon) and limit unhealthy, processed carbs, junk food, and sugar.

—CHIEN-WEI CHEN
NORMAN, OKLAHOMA
LBS. LOST 15

• • • • • • • •

**WHENEVER POSSIBLE,** eat lean meats that are not injected with hormones or antibiotics. Fish and poultry have been widely overlooked by low-carb consumers. Also, introduce good fats, such as olive oil or macadamia nut oil into your diet and be mindful of the amount of fiber and vegetables you consume. As long as it's working for you, you should eat more whole, unprocessed foods and grains and focus on making practical decisions in the foods you eat.

—LINDA LANGDON
VANCOUVER, BRITISH COLUMBIA, CANADA
LBS. LOST MORE THAN 100

• • • • • • • •

**I NO LONGER EAT "WHITE" FOODS,** such as white bread, white pasta, white potatoes, and white rice. I also eat foods that are as minimally processed as possible. So I especially avoid things like baked goods; they're made with white flour, and they're highly processed.

—LAURA VINCENT
SAN RAFAEL, CALIFORNIA
LBS. LOST 80

## SLIM STAT

Eating vegetables on a regular basis for two weeks helped volunteers reduce levels of stress-related molecules and boost their blood levels of vitamin C.

# SMALL EFFORT

To burn off the calories in one small chocolate chip cookie (50 calories), walk briskly for 10 minutes (for people of average weight) or longer (more than average weight).

**YOU HAVE TO EAT SOME CARBS** to build muscle. Any diet that tells you to throw out carbs completely is nuts. You need protein for muscles but the energy source that puts it all together is carbohydrates. So go ahead and eat that bread and don't feel guilty about it.

—*DAVID TRENT*
*WOODWORTH, OHIO*
*LBS. LOST 16*

. . . . . . . .

66 Instead of using salt, which makes you retain water, use spices that have a diuretic effect, like thyme, oregano, cayenne pepper, cinnamon, dill, and ginger. 99

—*CECILIA CARSON*
*COLUMBIA, MISSOURI*
*LBS. LOST 11*

. . . . . . . .

**Substitute one meal a day with a salad—any salad!**

—*K.B.*
*CHICAGO, ILLINOIS*

**I HAVE A GIRLFRIEND WHO IS CONSTANTLY** battling with her weight. I had her over for dinner once and realized that the major difference between the two of us was the amount of food we had stacked on our respective plates. Watching her eat and go back for repeat helpings, I clearly understood her battle with her weight. Yet, to her, the portions on her plate seemed normal and were never thought to be the cause of her problem.

—*OMO MISHA*
*NEW YORK, NEW YORK*

I MAKE SURE THAT I FOLLOW the five-a-day rule, and the easy way for me to do that is eating from the rainbow. If I eat at least one fruit and/or vegetable from each color group—red, purple, white, green, and yellow—then I know I am getting my five servings or more each day.

—KANDI KIZZIAH
ROCKY MOUNT, NORTH CAROLINA
LBS. LOST 158

. . . . . . . . .

STUDIES HAVE FOUND THAT PEOPLE will eat what you give them, never mind what a sensible portion is. Learn what the correct portion sizes are for your favorite foods. I find it helpful to eat on small plates, too. A small portion looks bigger on a small plate.

—KAT CARNEY
LOS ANGELES, CALIFORNIA
LBS. LOST 90

. . . . . . . . .

YOU HAVE TO WATCH FOR HIGH FAT content in foods, but understand that calories are more important. Some foods can be low in fat and high in calories. Ultimately, you have to burn off more calories each day than you consume. The number of fat grams in something can be misleading, but it's a good place to start.

—BRITTANY MELLOR
ZELIENOPLE, PENNSYLVANIA
LBS. LOST 15

A healthier alternative to pasta is spaghetti squash. I made it for my girlfriend and she didn't know the difference.

—TORREY MATUSEV
CANFIELD, OHIO
LBS. LOST 8

# MEDIUM EFFORT

To burn off the calories in a jelly-filled doughnut, you'd have to walk for one hour at a moderate pace (for people of average weight) or longer (more than average weight).

**CUT DOWN ON YOUR SALT INTAKE.** The most important thing I learned was how much sodium can affect your weight. I started using salt substitute, and it made a big difference in how much water weight I retained.

—*KAREN BUFFUM*
*ROUND ROCK, TEXAS*
*LBS. LOST 25*

• • • • • • • • •

**I USED TO EAT "REGULAR"** everything—regular mayonnaise, regular cheese, regular milk, etc. I tried fat-free things, but they taste like plastic to me. So I compromise and buy light or reduced-fat foods.

—*DIANE SZYMANSKI*
*SOUTH BEND, INDIANA*
*LBS. LOST 72*

• • • • • • • • •

**PEOPLE HAVE THE WRONG IDEA** about how to eat. The processed foods are the problem, not the natural fat in foods. If people gave up eating fast food and processed foods, they'd be surprised at how good a healthy diet is. Instead of eating low-fat crap, try eating something in its natural state.

—*NICK*
*DURHAM, NORTH CAROLINA*
*LBS. LOST 30*

• • • • • • • • •

**HEALTHY FOOD DOESN'T HAVE** to taste bad. Breaded, pan-seared, or baked fish is tasty and filling. Same goes for chicken. Salads, with the right salad dressing (in the right amount), can also be good. Find a vegetable you like to eat and have more of it. It's surprising how filling salads and veggies are. Whole wheat breads and brown rice are also tasty.

—*B.H.*
*SEATTLE, WASHINGTON*

I BEGAN TO DRINK EIGHT to ten glasses of water each day and I stopped eating chips, pretzels, popcorn, cake, etc. and ate only fruit, vegetables, protein, and very small amounts of carbs.

> —PATRICIA MICHENER
> WEST GROVE, PENNSYLVANIA
> LBS. LOST 146

• • • • • • • •

REMOVE COFFEE FROM YOUR DAILY DIET, as hard as that can be. If you absolutely can't do without it, you should wait an hour after eating before enjoying a cup of coffee or you will cut iron absorption in the body up to 40 percent.

> —BARRY DUGITA
> YOUNGSTOWN, PENNSYLVANIA
> LBS. LOST 14

• • • • • • • •

TAKE A SELECTION OF ANY vegetables (onions, mushrooms, carrots, cabbage, zucchini, eggplant, acorn squash, etc.), chop them up into smallish pieces, and season with whatever spices you like. Put it all in a roasting bag, tie it up, make a few small holes for the steam to escape, and bake it for about an hour until it's soft. It will last for about five days and is a hot and satisfying low-calorie meal.

> —MIRI GREIDI
> RA'ANANA, ISRAEL
> LBS. LOST 53

I always eat a banana first thing in the morning, and I always like it.

—J.L.
WOODLAND,
MARYLAND
LBS. LOST 16

# LARGE EFFORT

To burn off the calories in a fast-food meal of a double-patty cheeseburger, extra-large fries, and a 24 oz. soft drink (1,500 calories), you'd have to run two hours at a 10 min./mile pace (for people of average weight) or longer (more than average weight).

**I MIX MARSHMALLOWS** and Rice Krispies in the microwave. It's quick, delicious and much healthier than normal Rice Krispies treats because there's no butter involved.

—*KRISTEN HURD*
*TULSA, OKLAHOMA*
*LBS. LOST 20*

• • • • • • • •

**BEVERAGES CAN EITHER MAKE** or break your diet. Although juices are packed with nutrients, while dieting your better choice may be whole fruit. An apple will leave you feeling fuller while providing more fiber. Also, go very easy on the spirits. I love wine and like to think that it's made from grapes, so it must be good for me. But there are lots of calories in there. Once I kicked the wine from my diet I knew I could do it.

—*BEN NOBLE*
*YOUNGSTOWN, PENNSYLVANIA*
*LBS. LOST 21*

• • • • • • • •

**A FEW YEARS AGO,** I suffered from kidney failure and couldn't have any salt. I lost a lot of weight this way and also discovered many spices. Cooking with herbs and spices will add great flavor to your food and may help you lose weight. It worked for me!

—*ANONYMOUS*
*TORONTO, ONTARIO, CANADA*
*LBS. LOST 12*

• • • • • • • •

**WHEN I QUIT DRINKING I LOST WEIGHT** without even trying. Moving to a city probably helped too; you tend to walk more when you live in a city. But I stayed fat in the city until I gave up the booze.

—*JOE L.*
*BOSTON, MASSACHUSSETTS*
*LBS. LOST 20*

## IS IT THE FISH?

Japan consistently ranks among nations with the world's longest life spans, perhaps because of the country's common low-fat, fish-based diet.

# Work It: Getting in Shape Through Exercise (And Sex!)

E*xperts recommend we get 30 minutes of exercise three or more times a week. Sure, that's 4,680 minutes a year you could be sitting on the couch catching up on* Law and Order *reruns, but we're talking about your health here. In this chapter, you'll find dozens of tips and techniques to make the most of each and every one of those exercise minutes.*

**I RUN FIVE MILES ALMOST EVERY DAY,** and I don't even think about what I'm eating. If I want a damn cookie, I'm having a damn cookie.

—*BARB G.*
*PITTSBURGH, PENNSYLVANIA*
*LBS. LOST 9*

**HIT THE GYM... HARD!**

—*STEPHEN MACKAY*
*SAN FRANCISCO, CALIFORNIA*
*LBS. LOST 10*

**JOIN A GYM, GET A SUPPORT SYSTEM.** Join family-oriented places like the YMCA. They have a supportive training staff that can help.

—LARA LOEST
MILWAUKEE, WISCONSIN
LBS. LOST 15

· · · · · · · ·

" Work out in the morning. That way, you can't flake out at night when you come home from work and don't feel like making a trip to the gym. "

—F.V.
NEW YORK, NEW YORK
LBS. LOST 15

· · · · · · · ·

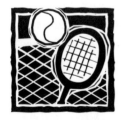

**THERE'S JUST NO GETTING AROUND** the fact that you need to watch what you eat and you need to exercise in order to lose weight. It's such a hellishly boring thing to tell people, but it's just the way it is. I exercise for at least an hour every morning—usually it's a five-mile run or lifting weights at the gym. There are many, many days I exercise with complete reluctance, but I have to say that I don't regret doing it afterward. It must trigger some sort of natural chemical-reaction voodoo in your body that just makes you feel like you're not the tub of lard you thought you were.

—EDGAR POMA
SAN FRANCISCO, CALIFORNIA
LBS. LOST 30

**FIND AN EXERCISE PROGRAM** that fits your lifestyle and don't be afraid to ease into it. I started with 10 minutes in the morning and 10 minutes in the evening. There are lots of exercise videos that are broken up into 10-minute exercise chunks. I find that if I start with just 10 minutes, I often feel so great that I work out for 20 or even 30 minutes.

> —KAT CARNEY
> LOS ANGELES, CALIFORNIA
> LBS. LOST *90*

* * * * * * * *

**MANY COMPANIES HAVE EXERCISE** facilities on-site or offer discounted memberships for fitness programs off-site. If you are one of those lucky people, you have to take advantage of it.

> —TOM T.
> COLUMBIANA, OHIO
> LBS. LOST *13*

* * * * * * * *

**SINCE I JUST NEEDED TO LOSE** a few pounds, I cut calories by simply switching to diet soft drinks and water, and I began walking briskly for 30 minutes on a treadmill, three or four mornings a week while watching the morning news. I also started eating breakfast. I found the light exercise in the morning and breakfast gave me more energy, curbed my appetite more during the day, and helped me sleep better at night.

> —NICKY G.
> OKLAHOMA CITY, OKLAHOMA
> LBS. LOST *15*

* * * * * * * *

**THERE IS A TRICK TO EXERCISING:** To reap the maximum benefits, you have to do it regularly, and you have to build up your weights slowly. You can't start working out with heavy weights.

> —ANONYMOUS
> NEW YORK, NEW YORK
> LBS. LOST *20*

## STAY STEADY

Sixty minutes of moderate-to vigorous-intensity activity on most days, while not exceeding caloric intake requirements, is recommended to manage weight.

# SEXERCISE

**THE BEST EXERCISE IS HAVING SEX.** You can tell your partner that if she wants you to lose weight she has to help you out. That way you both win.

> —*TONY COLAGUORI*
> *PITTSBURGH, PENNSYLVANIA*
> *LBS. LOST 20*

**PEOPLE WHO HAVE SEX REGULARLY REPORT** that they handle stress better. The release of climax will get even the most anxious lover totally relaxed, and you know you'll sleep better. And when you are more rested it's easier to exercise. And when you exercise you lose weight.

> —*FRANK CAPISO*
> *BOARDMAN, OHIO*
> *LBS. LOST 8*

**IS THERE A BETTER DIET EXERCISE PROGRAM THAN SEX?** If so, I want to hear about it.

> —*PAM SASSER*
> *WHEELING, WEST VIRGINIA*
> *LBS. LOST 15*

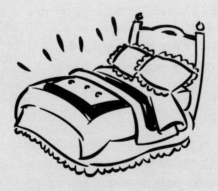

**WOULD YOU RATHER RUN 75 MILES** or have sex three times a week for one year? Both burn about the same calories, but one is decidedly more pleasurable than the other. Regular sex—which burns approximately 150 calories in a half-hour—is regular exercise. You'll have all the same benefits of spending that time in the gym, including improved circulation and lower cholesterol. Trust me, my son is a doctor.

> —CHAD MORTON
> POLAND, OHIO
> LBS. LOST 11

. . . . . . . . .

**I CAN'T THINK OF ANY BETTER EXCUSE** to give your wife if she doesn't want to have sex with you. If you tell her it's so that you can be healthier and live longer, what's she going to say to that? I bet she won't be faking any headaches when you come to her with that line.

> —DALE JENNINGS
> FROSTBURG, MARYLAND
> LBS. LOST 12

. . . . . . . . .

**WHEN I STARTED MY DIET,** my doctor told me that people who had sex once or twice per week enjoyed higher levels of an antibody that helps fend off illness. In other words sex keeps you from getting sick. And it keeps you healthier. I'm all for that.

> —BETSY ANDERSEN
> CANFIELD, OHIO
> LBS. LOST 18

. . . . . . . . .

**SEX IS DOCTOR-APPROVED** as one of the best forms of an all-body workout. You're working up a sweat, you aren't watching the clock (hopefully), and it burns tons of calories.

> —KRISTEN HURD
> TULSA, OKLAHOMA
> LBS. LOST 20

**A** FRIEND TOLD ME ABOUT THIS STUDY that I'm not sure I believe, but I hope it's true. She said a study of 1,000 men found that those who had at least two orgasms per week had half the death rate of those who indulged less than once a month. It said sex can make you look younger, too. Men and women who reported having sex an average of four times per week looked approximately ten years younger than they really were. To tell you the truth, if I look ten years younger I don't care if I'm fat.

—*SUE LASKY*
*POLAND, OHIO*
*LBS. LOST 17*

• • • • • • • •

**SEX DEFINITELY** counts as exercise.

—*J.S.*
*NEW YORK, NEW YORK*

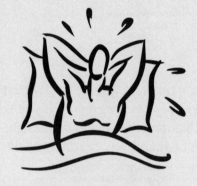

**BUY A HEART RATE MONITOR.** I had hit a plateau in my weight loss and was frustrated because I had cut out junk food and walked every day, but my progress was stalled. After I got the monitor, I discovered that I wasn't getting my heart rate into the fat-burning zone or training zone. It motivated me to work harder and thus get maximum value for the walking time. I'm off the plateau now.

—*ANONYMOUS*
*NEW YORK, NEW YORK*
*LBS. LOST 17*

66 Keep active. Playing sports is always fun, but if you're not an athlete, simply walking around or doing chores regularly are good ways to keep fat from building up. 99

—*JERMAINE B. WILLIAMS*

**I TRY TO WALK EACH NIGHT AFTER SUPPER.** Besides the walking itself helping me lose weight, it gets me out of the house at a critical snacking time. My wife walks with me, so it's a great time for us to talk and reconnect each day. We take our dog along, too, so it gets him some exercise, and it makes him happy. We have a standard two-mile loop that we walk around our neighborhood.

—*MICHAEL REICH*
*HELLERTOWN, PENNSYLVANIA*
*LBS. LOST 7*

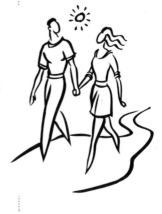

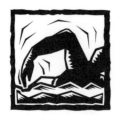

**TO KEEP YOURSELF FROM GETTING TIRED** of working out and to work different muscle groups it's good to do different things on different days. I jog three days a week, swim twice a week, and bike every now and then. I think if you just jog every day that would get old quick.

—*M.E.S.*
*CARNEGIE, PENNSYLVANIA*
LBS. LOST *8*

• • • • • • • • •

**EXERCISE IS SO IMPORTANT,** but it has to be consistent. I used to exercise for a month, then stop. But this last time, I made exercise a part of my life. I began by just walking for 20 minutes three times a week on my treadmill. Gradually, I increased it to 30 minutes. About a month later, I started doing free weights at home. Then I took an indoor spinning class. I realized that I love cycling, so I bought a road bike. Today, I cycle 100 to 120 miles a week in season, I teach a yoga class at the YMCA seven days a week, I do weight training three times a week, and I teach a class introducing women to weight training.

—*JOAN RAINWATER*
*WATERVILLE, OHIO*
LBS. LOST *37*

**Work out to music. When I run on the treadmill I get bored if I don't have my headset on with a good CD.**

—*F.V.*
*NEW YORK,*
*NEW YORK*
LBS. LOST *15*

• • • • • • • • •

**I NEVER REALLY TRIED EXERCISING.** It wasn't until I started rowing on the college crew team that I started to appreciate my body's strengths and what it could do. Being part of an organized sport, interacting with other people, and discovering my competitiveness helped immensely. It took my focus off clothing size and what I was eating and put it onto a larger purpose: contributing to a team effort.

—*ALANA WATKINS*
*DENVER, COLORADO*
LBS. LOST *25*

**I PRACTICE YOGA,** and I think it is the best form of exercise. It is an exercise for the brain as well as the body. And for those of you who want to see results, your body will look great. Just take a look at your local yoga instructor. I guarantee you she or he has a great-looking body.

—*ALME BLAIR*

• • • • • • • •

**WHEN IT COMES TO EXERCISING,** I don't think that it is worth doing if you don't really push yourself. When you are doing crunches, for instance, you aren't really getting much done if your muscles don't ache afterwards.

—*ANONYMOUS*
*NEW YORK, NEW YORK*
*LBS. LOST 25*

• • • • • • • •

**EXERCISE EARLY IN THE MORNING,** right after you wake up. I got up at 6 a.m. five days a week and worked out for an hour. It boosted my metabolism for the entire day and left me feeling much more energetic and productive.

—*LENNARD HAYNES SR.*
*HOUSTON, TEXAS*
*LBS. LOST 40*

• • • • • • • •

**THE GYM IS A HALF HOUR** from my house. During the week, it's convenient because it's close to my office, but on weekends, it's a pain in the neck to get there, so I work out at home. Specifically, I love doing tapes: *Tae Bo, Pilates,* the old *Eight-Minute Arms, Thighs and Buns.* There's a really good collection called *Slim in Six,* which is a mix of cardio and toning. It is possible to get a good workout outside the gym.

—*JAYME*
*O'FALLON, MISSOURI*

**HEY, I CAN DO THAT!**

The average, 150-pound person burns 360 calories a night while sleeping.

# WHY EXERCISE?

**WALKING CHANGED MY BODY** so much. Once I started to see those changes, it made me so happy I felt a boost to keep doing it. Combining walking with eating right produced amazing results.

>—*DIANE SZYMANSKI*
>*SOUTH BEND, INDIANA*
>*LBS. LOST 72*

. . . . . . . .

**BESIDES ACTUALLY HELPING ME LOSE WEIGHT,** exercise makes me feel better. Feeling better keeps me from emotional eating and craving comfort foods. I joined a gym about a month and a half ago, and I exercise there at least three times a week.

>—*CAROL*
>*EASTON, PENNSYLVANIA*
>*LBS. LOST 40*

. . . . . . . .

**EXERCISING HELPS ME CURB MY SWEET TOOTH:** I'm a sweetaholic. But when I exercise, the time I spend is an investment, and I don't want to undo it all with snacks.

>—*KATIE*
>*OREM, UTAH*
>*LBS. LOST 45*

. . . . . . . .

**I EXERCISE MY WAY OUT OF THINGS** so I can enjoy eating and continue to eat all my favorite foods!

>—*ANONYMOUS*
>*SAN FRANCISCO, CALIFORNIA*
>*LBS. LOST 8*

. . . . . . . .

**EXERCISE IS CRITICAL IF YOU DON'T WANT** hanging skin. I started exercising before I had gastric-bypass surgery. Now I go to the gym six days a week, and I don't have any hanging skin—none!

>—*LAURA SIGHINOLFI*
>*BOCA RATON, FLORIDA*
>*LBS. LOST 150*

**PEOPLE DON'T REALIZE THAT WALKING** is good exercise. Just because you aren't sweating doesn't mean that you aren't getting a valid workout. When you have to go somewhere that is 20 blocks away, or a mile down the road, walk. Every little bit counts, and before you know it, you'll be thinner and have more energy!

—*ANGELA CHANG*

* * * * * * * *

**THERE IS NO EASY WAY TO GET IN SHAPE,** to look and feel good. The only way is to work at it. I run a few miles a day, at least five days a week. I set my alarm clock for 6 a.m. every morning and put my workout clothes by the side of the bed. That way, I can get up, put them on, and be out the door!

—*ROCHELLE ADAMES*

* * * * * * * *

**NO ONE'S ASKING YOU** to run a marathon. Take the stairs to your office (within reason, of course). A quick jog in the morning or in the evening will do wonders. And if you don't like jogging, try walking, or swimming. Better yet, take up a sport you've been meaning to learn— rock climbing, tennis, martial arts. Even a half hour a day of exercise will help; it'll boost your metabolism and make you feel better.

—*BOB HOLDEN*
*NEW YORK, NEW YORK*

* * * * * * * *

**FIND SOMETHING THAT INVOLVES** getting your heart rate elevated. Walk, play tennis, swim: Whatever you like to do and *can* do three or four times a week for about 45 minutes will get the job done.

—*KEITH MCCARTHY*
*PITTSBURGH, PENNSYLVANIA*
LBS. LOST 15

Keep your body off-kilter. I think if you keep doing the same exercise day after day, your body gets used to it and it isn't helping as much.

—*ANNMARIE PEARSON*
*GIG HARBOR, WASHINGTON*
LBS. LOST 68

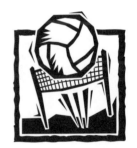

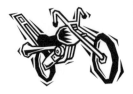

**EXERCISE HELPS TREMENDOUSLY.** I had a stationary bicycle in a room with a TV. It was just a simple, no-frills bike, but it really burned the weight off. I biked for one hour each night. When I neared my weight-loss goal, I was in such good shape that I could have even kept going after an hour!

—*JENNIFER*
*READING, PENNSYLVANIA*
*LBS. LOST 70*

. . . . . . . .

*"* Don't look at exercising as a chore or negative aspect of your day. Develop the attitude that it's your time for yourself to do something positive and healthy in your day. *"*

—*ERIN*
*FRANKLIN, MASSACHUSETTS*
*LBS. LOST 40*

. . . . . . . .

**I COULDN'T HAVE LOST THE WEIGHT** without exercising. Three days a week, I do one hour of Tae Bo and one hour of weights. Then, two days a week I use the treadmill during my favorite daytime show, *Days of Our Lives*. I walk while the show is on and jog during the commercials.

—*ANNMARIE PEARSON*
*GIG HARBOR, WASHINGTON*
*LBS. LOST 68*

**ESPECIALLY IF YOU HAVE KIDS,** think of ways to incorporate exercise into your everyday routine. When my daughter started daycare, I bought a trailer for my bicycle. Now I bike about two hours to take her to daycare.

—KRISTEN
BETHLEHEM, PENNSYLVANIA

• • • • • • • •

**HOW DO YOU FIND TIME TO EXERCISE?** I never find time to exercise; I have to *make* time to exercise. I enjoy exercising because it clears my mind and it is a nice way to get out of the house. I make time to do it, and it becomes a part of my daily routine.

—MIA KIRCHMEIER
REDMOND, WASHINGTON
LBS. LOST 25

• • • • • • • •

**JOIN A GYM** and get a personal trainer. He'll be waiting for you, so you have no excuse not to work out.

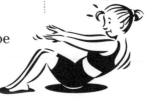

—S.A.
LAKE FOREST, CALIFORNIA
LBS. LOST 15

# JOG THROUGH

The *Dallas Morning News* tallied up the number of calories people could burn if they replaced several "convenient" activities, such as driving through a "drive-through" window, with their more active counterparts, such as walking into the store. Together, they added up to 8,800 calories worth of missed physical activity opportunities each month, or the amount of activity needed to burn off 2.5 pounds of fat.

# CALORIES: WHERE DO THEY GO?

Seventy percent of the calories you consume are burned on a daily basis for what we call your metabolic requirements; in other words, the energy to keep your body alive, the fuel to keep your heart beating, your lungs expanding, your brain functioning, and your liver and kidneys filtering.

Twenty percent of the calories go to what is called activities of daily living, which includes the energy needed to make your bed, drive your car, work on your computer, or brush your teeth.

Ten percent of the calories go to something called thermogenesis—the calories it takes to break down the calories you just ate.

The key to weight loss is increasing the percentage of calories that you burn off with physical activity. Whether you exercise, play a sport, or are physically active, the more you move your body, the more calories your body will require and burn.

**NO MATTER HOW MUCH** you enjoy something, you don't want to do it every day. You should choose an activity that you can stand, but don't force yourself to do it all the time. If you don't like to walk or run, then try swimming or biking. The key is finding something that you can stomach.

—*MATT MARSHALL*
*EVANS CITY, PENNSYLVANIA*
*LBS. LOST 11*

" Find an *activity* you enjoy—
nobody enjoys *exercise*. "

—*DANIEL COLLINS*
*COCKEYSVILLE, MARYLAND*
*LBS. LOST 56*

**I'VE NEVER BEEN GOOD** at consistently exercising, but the one thing that I enjoy is riding my bike with my husband. A lot of times, I'm not motivated to go, but when we get back from a bike ride I realize that I'm not hungry and we just have something small for supper.

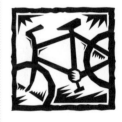

—*AMY*
*ALBURTIS, PENNSYLVANIA*

**GET INTO A ROUTINE OF EXERCISE,** and you won't have to worry about dieting. I lost the most weight I have ever lost, and kept it off, by walking every day for a half hour. I walked 15 minutes to a coffee shop and treated myself to a cup of coffee and then I walked home.

—*LENAN SHELTON*
*AUSTIN, TEXAS*
*LBS. LOST 25*

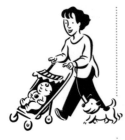

**I CAN THROW MY KID** in the stroller and take care of an errand or two by walking to the grocery store.

—*ANONYMOUS*
*LOS ANGELES, CALIFORNIA*
*LBS. LOST 20*

. . . . . . . .

**I DECIDED TO TRY RUNNING** in the mornings. I live in a beautiful place and get home from work when the sun is down. By running in the mornings, I was able to enjoy the surroundings and lose weight at the same time. It gave me energy the rest of the day and made me feel less trapped in my office.

—*JEFFREY TOCKMAN*
*SAN FRANCISCO, CALIFORNIA*
*LBS. LOST 15*

. . . . . . . .

**I DON'T GO TO THE GYM;** I have one in my house. It consists of a full-size treadmill, free weights and a modified weight bench. I really like working out on my own, wearing what I like, and not having to drive anywhere. Plus, I'm 40 and have no desire to be around a bunch of buff 20-year-olds.

—*DEBBIE REDDEN-BRUNELLO*
*TEMECULA, CALIFORNIA*
*LBS. LOST 30*

# GET MOVING

Regular, leisure-time physical activity is defined as light or moderate activity five times or more per week for 30 minutes or more each time, and/or vigorous activity three times or more per week for 20 minutes or more each time. It's no wonder less than 33% of American adults are doing it!

# MORE ON METABOLISM: WHERE DID THE MUSCLE GO?

There are two major ways we lose muscle. One way is through the natural aging process. Beginning in our mid-to-late 30s, we tend to lose perhaps as much as a half-pound of muscle each year. Over the next 10 years, we may lose up to five pounds of muscle mass just through aging. At almost 50 calories per pound, that is 250 fewer calories your body will burn in a day. Thus you will gain weight unless you make adjustments to your exercise and diet. This is why exercise to maintain muscle or minimize muscle loss, is vital throughout your life, and especially as you age.

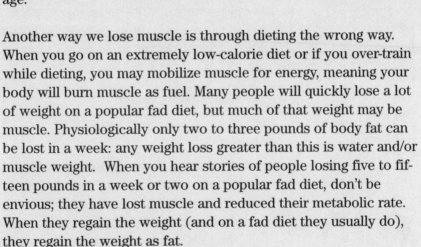

Another way we lose muscle is through dieting the wrong way. When you go on an extremely low-calorie diet or if you over-train while dieting, you may mobilize muscle for energy, meaning your body will burn muscle as fuel. Many people will quickly lose a lot of weight on a popular fad diet, but much of that weight may be muscle. Physiologically only two to three pounds of body fat can be lost in a week: any weight loss greater than this is water and/or muscle weight.  When you hear stories of people losing five to fifteen pounds in a week or two on a popular fad diet, don't be envious; they have lost muscle and reduced their metabolic rate. When they regain the weight (and on a fad diet they usually do), they regain the weight as fat.

**YOU HAVE TO DO INTERVAL TRAINING** or you won't get the maximum benefits out of your workout. Try sprinting on the treadmill, and then jog. One day, do yoga, and the next day do cycling. Keep your body tired and do new activities to lose as much weight as possible.

—*G.L.*
*NEW YORK, NEW YORK*
*LBS. LOST 15*

## YEAH, I CAN DO THAT!

Sitting there, reading this book, you're burning 114 calories per hour (for an average, 150-pound person).

**PEOPLE GET BURNED OUT** by the tremendous exertion of running all the time. You can do your body just as much good by walking, and it's a lot more enjoyable. If you jog five days a week, start doing brisk walking on one or two of those days instead. Also, start walking to places that you usually drive to. There is a small market near my house that I used to always drive to. Now I walk, weather permitting. It only takes about seven minutes to get there, but I know that I'm burning calories that would have stayed on my body in the past.

—*BOB*
*PITTSBURGH, PENNSYLVANIA*
*LBS. LOST 17*

**I'M PART OF A WEIGHT-LOSS GROUP** at work. We exercise together, and that has helped a lot. I like to exercise, but doing it by myself has far less appeal. We buddy up to go for walks. I find it's safer that way, too. Our group has tried different types of exercise, too, so we don't get bored. Our staple is walking, but we've tried step aerobics, Pilates, ball and band workouts, and free weights. One member of our group brought in a salsa aerobics tape: That was a lot of fun!

—*DAPHNE*
*OREM, UTAH*
*LBS. LOST 47*

**YOU HAVE TO BE SELFISH SOMETIMES.** Go to the gym instead of staying late at work or volunteering at your kids' school. Make time to sit down for a relaxing lunch instead of multi-tasking. If the President can find time to exercise an hour a day, so can you.

—*JESSICA ROTHMAN*
*NEW YORK, NEW YORK*
LBS. LOST *25*

• • • • • • • •

**ROUTINE IS EVERYTHING WHEN** it comes to exercising. I find it harder to exercise every other day or two to three times a week than exercising daily. If I go to the gym three times in a row, it becomes part of my routine and I remain consistent and will continue to work out. If I skip days, it's harder for me to get into the swing of things.

—*G.P.*
*IOWA CITY, IOWA*

• • • • • • • •

**WITH A NEW BABY,** I think it's easiest to work out at home. Sure, I might have liked to join a gym, but then I would have needed to get a babysitter for my son. So instead I simply did push-ups, sit-ups, and toning exercises at home.

—*GWEN*
*HELLERTOWN, PENNSYLVANIA*
LBS. LOST *47*

• • • • • • • •

**TO LOSE ONE POUND YOU NEED** to burn off about 3,500 more calories than you take in. It doesn't matter if those calories come in cookies, bananas, or meat. Learn to count your calories and then burn off more than you eat. Heck, even breathing burns off some calories, and we can all do that pretty well.

—*TOM BUFORD*
*BOARDMAN, OHIO*
LBS. LOST *5*

Always stretch first. I got on a treadmill without warming up and pulled a tendon in my ankle. By the time it healed I was out of the habit of going to the gym.

—*SUE SIFFORD*
*SIKESTON, MISSOURI*
LBS. LOST *15*

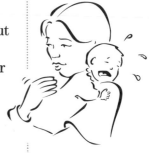

# LET'S GET ORIGINAL

**HERE'S A GREAT EXERCISE ROUTINE** I learned in the Army. Take a deck of cards. Flip the cards over one by one and do the number of pushups or sit-ups that corresponds to the number on the cards. You could do pushups for red cards and sit-ups for black cards, for instance. So if the first card you flip over is the three of hearts, do three pushups. All face cards are worth ten, so if you flip over the king of spades, do ten sit-ups.

—*ANONYMOUS*
*HELLERTOWN, PENNSYLVANIA*
*LBS. LOST 13*

• • • • • • • •

**TAKE A DANCE CLASS.** I enjoy belly dancing. I recently moved across the country, from Massachusetts to California. Fortunately I found a dance studio where I take classes. Belly dancing is much more popular in California. An extra bonus is I'm getting to know other people in the area.

—*LAURA VINCENT*
*SAN RAFAEL, CALIFORNIA*
*LBS. LOST 80*

• • • • • • • •

**I NEVER EXERCISE, BUT I DO HOUSEWORK**—picking up loads of laundry, mopping and vacuuming the floors. Also, when my child was little, I would lift him over my head.

—*NANCY*
*NICEVILLE, FLORIDA*

• • • • • • • •

**GET A JOB WHERE YOU WORK ON YOUR FEET.** I've lost about 15 pounds working in retail, where I run around getting shipments, helping customers and answering the phones.

—*T.V.*
*SAN ANTONIO, TEXAS*
*LBS. LOST 15*

**FOR THE PAST NINE YEARS,** I've exercised in the bathroom. I close the door, turn on the air vent, and do about 20 minutes' worth of sit-ups and leg lifts. It's great, because it's peaceful, quiet, and well decorated, and nobody interrupts me. That's the secret to making an exercise routine stick: Find a place that you enjoy going to.

—*P.O.*
*NEW BRUNSWICK, NEW JERSEY*
*LBS. LOST 50*

**GO OUT DANCING! I SWEAR, WHEN I LEFT MY HUSBAND** I went out dancing two or three times a week, and it was the best exercise ever! You get all sweaty without experiencing that thing that happens when you jog—you think you'd rather just be fat than run one more step. I lost so much weight. I still do that if I feel like I'm getting fat, especially in the winter when outside exercise is harder to pull off. I make dates with my friends to go out dancing instead of to movies or restaurants.

—*AMY*
*DURHAM, NORTH CAROLINA*
*LBS. LOST 25*

**TWO FRIENDS ASKED ME TO JOIN THEM** in dancing to music tapes for 30 minutes without stopping, a few times a week. We play The Supremes and Cher. I do the twist. We are all over 50, and we love to talk about where we were at the time a particular song came out. In just a few weeks, I have lost 15 pounds.

—*S.B.*
*KERALA, INDIA*
*LBS. LOST 15*

**I'M NOT ONE OF THOSE PEOPLE** who loves to exercise, but a friend of mine does. She drags me out to walk every day. "Come on, you can do it," she says to encourage me. It really helps get me outside to walk, which has helped me lose weight.

—*TERESA*
  *SALEM, UTAH*
  *LBS. LOST 7*

• • • • • • • •

**WHEN I HIT MIDDLE AGE,** my pants got tighter! Even though I have five kids to run after, I found that I needed to add exercise to my life. My goal was to lose five pounds, and I lost 17. I walk in the morning and run on my treadmill at night.

—*LIZA*
  *OREM, UTAH*
  *LBS. LOST 17*

• • • • • • • •

**I CAN'T AFFORD TO JOIN A GYM NOW,** but I walk and use exercise videos. I have five-pound weights at home, and I use them regularly.

—*MELISSA WASHINGTON*
  *BROOKLYN, NEW YORK*
  *LBS. LOST 20*

• • • • • • • •

**EXERCISE-WALKING WITH FRIENDS** is the best way to make myself get up and get out of the house. It motivates me tremendously. My pace is quicker, and I learn so much from the conversations we have while walking; it's like therapy. The other thing I love is my Digi-Walker. It's a pedometer that captures steps; you don't even have to set it. It monitors how active you are. Ten thousand steps per day is the equivalent of five miles, and as long as I do that I can eat a normal amount of food and not gain weight.

—*ANONYMOUS*
  *WAKEFIELD, NEW HAMPSHIRE*
  *LBS. LOST 10*

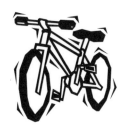

**I PREFER TO GET MY EXERCISE OUTDOORS.** I'll take windsurfing, biking, and swimming over working out on a treadmill any day!

> —ANONYMOUS
> NEW YORK, NEW YORK
> LBS. LOST 20

• • • • • • • •

**THERE ARE REALLY FUN WAYS** to lose weight if you don't enjoy the gym. Go outside and shoot hoops with a friend or go for a long walk in the city. You don't have to lift weights to work out your body.

> —F.V.
> NEW YORK, NEW YORK
> LBS. LOST 15

• • • • • • • •

**IF YOU WALK, TRY WALKING** just a little faster. You burn off about 80 more calories an hour just by walking three miles an hour compared to two miles an hour. That's just a little bump up in speed, but to get 80 more calories off your fat butt is well worth the extra effort.

> —BERNIE VERONA
> BOARDMAN, OHIO
> LBS. LOST 9

• • • • • • • •

**THE BEST THING WHEN DIETING** is to do exercises you like, not necessarily those that are going to burn the most calories the quickest. I've tried to force myself to run because it burns the most calories. But I hate running; it makes me miserable. However, I love taking long walks. Taking walks may not burn off as many calories as running, but I know I'll take a long walk once a day. If I kept my mind set on running, I'd never burn anything off because I'd never get myself to run as often.

> —J.H.
> GLENDALE HEIGHTS, ILLINOIS
> LBS. LOST 20

## AND I'M ALREADY DOING THAT!

The average, 150-pound person burns 81 minutes watching *Lost* (or any one-hour TV show for that matter—we just happen to like *Lost*).

I used to leave a picture of Tammy Lee Webb (an aerobics guru) on my treadmill while I jogged. It made me feel supervised!

—*Anne Smalley*
*Woodbury,*
*New Jersey*
*lbs. lost 10*

**If you listen to a Walkman** while you are walking, try a book on tape. You become engrossed in the stories and forget that you're actually getting a workout. If I don't listen to the tape except when I'm walking, I really look forward to my next walk, so I can find out what happens next in the story. I never looked forward to the walks before I started doing that.

—*Shari Berg*
*Ellerslie, Maryland*
*lbs. lost 8*

• • • • • • • •

**Run away from your problem!** The best thing that you can do to lose weight is run, but boy, is it hard! If running bores you to tears, just make a game out of it: Walk a block, then run a block. Or jog on a treadmill and when it gets to 2:00, sprint as fast as you can for 30 seconds, then go back to your normal pace, or even walk if you have to. Not only does this make the time go fast, but it increases your metabolism and your endurance more than jogging alone.

—*Samantha Phillips*
*Atlanta, Georgia*
*lbs. lost 25*

• • • • • • • •

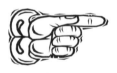

**As you get in better shape,** you have to increase your workout. You burn more calories as a fat person than as a skinny person doing the same thing; I guess it's because you have more to burn. I started out as a walker, but as it got easier I didn't feel I was accomplishing as much. I started jogging and eventually I started running. I burn about four times the calories running than I did walking for the same period of time. But you have to walk before you can run.

—*Greg Devries*
*Poland, Ohio*
*lbs. lost 22*

# MAKE YOUR OWN MOVES

*If a treadmill just reminds you of your job, find other ways to burn off some calories. Here is some creative thinking from others.*

**MY DAD HAS ALWAYS COLLECTED FIREWOOD** because we camp so much. He has a mechanical wood splitter, but I refuse to use it. Instead, once or twice a week, I'll spend two to three hours chopping wood by hand. It's an excellent workout and a great stress reliever. What better way to get your anger out than with an ax?

> —ANTHONY MANUEL
> KINDER, LOUISIANA
> *LBS. LOST 15*

- - - - - - - - -

**I PLAY TENNIS FOUR TO FIVE TIMES** a week for an hour and a half each time. It's a phenomenal sport. You have fun, you run your ass off, and you don't even realize you're doing it. It'll take weight off you like that. Of course, we're talking about singles tennis here, not doubles: Doubles is for wusses.

> —RICH
> ANN ARBOR, MICHIGAN
> *LBS. LOST 20*

- - - - - - - - -

**GOING TO THE GYM ALWAYS INTIMIDATED ME;** there were all these women in their perfect clothes with their perfect makeup. I started thinking about what I really liked to do. The answer was rollerblading. I figured it was great exercise, and I had access to a park with a good path. Now I look forward to doing it, and it's hard to obsess about your hair when you're wearing a helmet.

> —M.G.
> BELLEVILLE, ILLINOIS
> *LBS. LOST 25*

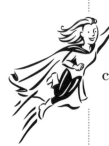

**RUNNING IS ABSOLUTELY THE BEST EXERCISE** you can do. My body was at its natural weight when I slowly started training for a marathon with my friend. About six weeks into our regimen, I had lost 13 pounds even though I was eating more than ever. Running burns so many calories. It's the best way to drop pounds.

—*ALANA WATKINS*
*DENVER, COLORADO*
*LBS. LOST 25*

· · · · · · · ·

**LEARN TO PLAY TENNIS,** or if you already know how, get out there and play! Tennis burns about twice the calories compared to walking, for the same period of time. And it's much more fun. I started playing only for diet reasons, but now I'm hooked. I love the sport.

—*ELMER GANTZ*
*POLAND, OHIO*
*LBS. LOST 17*

I try to walk as much as possible. If I can avoid driving, I do. I walk 25 minutes to work every day.

—*K.B.*
*CHICAGO, ILLINOIS*

· · · · · · · ·

**BUILDING MUSCLE HELPS** you burn more calories and allows any diet you may try to be more effective than restricting or monitoring food content alone.

—*D.N.*
*EUREKA SPRINGS, ARKANSAS*
*LBS. LOST 30*

· · · · · · · ·

**FENCING HELPS ME LOSE** and maintain weight. I've been a competitive fencer for 18 years and currently hold a C2 ranking in foil. Because I enjoy the sport and the people I meet through competition and the club I helped found, Chesapeake Fencing, I keep coming back and staying active. Fencing is definitely not boring!

—*DANIEL COLLINS*
*COCKEYSVILLE, MARYLAND*
*LBS. LOST 56*

IF YOU'RE A JOGGER OR A WALKER, don't go to a track. I used to do that, but it's too boring. Walk in your own neighborhood, but take a different route each day. You'll get distracted by looking at places you are used to seeing in the car but not on foot. It takes your mind off the work.

—CARL COOKE
CUMBERLAND, MARYLAND
LBS. LOST 10

I SAW AN AD FOR A MARATHON that was nine weeks away, and I decided to go for it. It helps to have tangible goals that you can achieve. Each time you reach your goal, you'll be inspired to set the bar even higher.

—JEFFREY TOCKMAN
SAN FRANCISCO, CALIFORNIA
LBS. LOST 15

I heard that even when we sleep we are burning calories. That's my kind of workout.

—WALKER EDWARDS
CANFIELD, OHIO
LBS. LOST 7

JOIN A HEALTH CLUB. I've found that once I spend the exorbitant entrance fee I'm too cheap to blow it off. I know I'll use the club because I don't want my money to go to waste. And I've found that when you are in there with all those people who are in shape, it is extra motivation for you.

—BILLY TRAMPER
FROSTBURG, MARYLAND
LBS. LOST 12

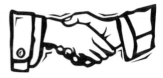

WHEN I BEGAN REGULARLY WORKING OUT, I realized that I slept better and felt more energized. I came to the conclusion that I am also more positive and have a better outlook on myself, as well as on life in general. I now try to focus on feeling peaceful, growing as a person, and being the best person I can be.

—CLAUDIA
MISSOURI
LBS. LOST 25

# MAN'S BEST EXERCISE PARTNER

**GET A DOG.** Initially, she was what got me out of the house and running. I don't think that now, nine years later, I need her. It's become enough of a routine for me that it's an ingrained habit. But she sure was a great motivator.

> —DAVID HUBBELL
> KIRKLAND, WASHINGTON
> LBS. LOST 50

• • • • • • • • •

**I WASN'T ABLE TO EXERCISE** when I first started my diet, due to a back injury. But after a few months, I was able to start walking each day with my dog. I think that adding exercise to my weight-loss program was the final change that really helped me get to my goal weight.

> —JENNIFER K.
> SHEBOYGAN, WISCONSIN
> LBS. LOST 22

• • • • • • • • •

**MY DOG, WINSTON,** is a tremendous motivator for me. We really walk every day, usually several times a day. But I'm careful to tailor our walks to the Chicago weather. On a nice, summer day, we might walk for more than an hour. But when it's 20 below, we go out for short periods of time several times a day.

> —KATHLEEN O'DEKIRK
> CHICAGO, ILLINOIS
> LBS. LOST 13

**I DID WHAT A LOT OF PEOPLE** do when they want to lose weight: I tried to stop eating so much. But pretty soon it seemed like I couldn't eat anything without it showing up on the scales. It was scary. What saved me is that a dog adopted me. This was a big, 80-pound animal that needed lots of exercise. I ended up walking him twice a day and before I knew it, I'd lost a few pounds. That inspired me to take a yoga class, which firmed up my body, and I lost a few more pounds. Within six months, I had lost 30 pounds, and I've kept it off for several years now.

—*JOANNE WOLFE*
*NESKOWIN, OREGON*
*LBS. LOST 30*

**I TOOK PART IN A STUDY** that compared people who exercised with their dogs to people who exercised without dogs to see who would lose more weight. When the study began, they gave us pedometers and the goal to walk 10,000 steps a day. I was surprised to find that in a normal day, I walk only 3,000 to 4,000 steps. Most people don't realize how little we move! During the year-long study, I began focusing on the 10,000 steps, and my dog, Spats, and I walked just about every day. It really helped.

—*ROSEANN LOCASCIO*
*CHICAGO, ILLINOIS*
*LBS. LOST 30*

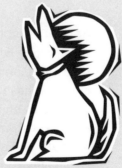

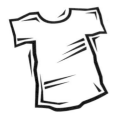

**WHEN I LOST 36 POUNDS** I joined a gym. But I have to admit I didn't actually go until I had lost 60. When I had lost 100 pounds, I made it a habit. At first I walked on the treadmill and took aerobics classes. Now I do cardio boxing. It's a great way to work out aggression!

> —*KARA*
> *CHICAGO, ILLINOIS*
> *LBS. LOST 217*

• • • • • • • •

**IF I DON'T EXERCISE ONE DAY,** that's fine. But I make sure I'm careful about what I eat and I definitely go the next day. Never let two days turn into three or four because you will be undoing all the hard work you've done.

> —*STEPHANIE CONE*
> *MONROE, IOWA*
> *LBS. LOST 20*

• • • • • • • •

**FIND A CONVENIENT TIME TO WALK.** When I was losing weight after my daughters were born, I walked each day on my lunch hour with some friends from work.

> —*DONNA*
> *ALLENTOWN, PENNSYLVANIA*
> *LBS. LOST 32*

• • • • • • • •

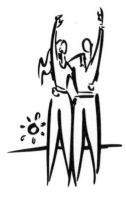

**I GOT A PERSONAL TRAINER FOR PILATES,** whom I have to pay whether I show up or not. I am, therefore, motivated to show up; she is not cheap. It has toned my body and given me muscle awareness and control. It has also helped enormously with range of movement, balance, strength and everyday aches and pains. In short, it changes your body shape, and mine certainly needed changing!

> —*SHARON LONDON*
> *SAN FRANCISCO, CALIFORNIA*
> *LBS. LOST 18*

**THERE HAS TO BE SOME OTHER REASON** to exercise besides losing weight for it to work and for you to keep it up. You have to enjoy it. It has to mean something to you. If walking is your alone time that you really enjoy, that might work. If you can focus on something other than your weight, you're more likely to stick to it.

—*MARY*
*NEW YORK, NEW YORK*
LBS. LOST *7*

- - - - - - - - -

**THE WAY I STICK TO MY WORKOUTS** is by keeping the expectations low each time I go in. The toughest part of any workout is just getting to the gym, so if I tell myself beforehand that it will be a short workout, there's much less dread involved. Once I'm there, I usually end up working out longer than I planned, thanks to this ritualistic cycle of self-deceit. I'd recommend it to anybody.

—*J.A.*
*IOWA CITY, IOWA*
LBS. LOST *15*

- - - - - - - - -

**MY FAVORITE FORM OF EXERCISE** is the Curves program, which combines toning and cardio workouts, all in one half-hour session. The results and the weight loss are not immediate, but the boost in energy and stamina is!

—*JOANE DAVIS*

- - - - - - - - -

**GIVE ROLLERBLADING A CHANCE.** I had never done this before I started dieting. I get too bored with jogging and walking, and there isn't a swimming pool near me. Rollerblading is lots of fun, and I assume I'm burning lots of calories because it's a real workout.

—*ANONYMOUS*
*CORRIGANVILLE, MARYLAND*
LBS. LOST *5*

Everybody needs an HPT: Hottie Personal Trainer. I have one and it helps tremendously with motivation and accountability. Looking at him doesn't hurt either!

—*S.H.*
*MINOT,*
*NORTH DAKOTA*
LBS. LOST *20*

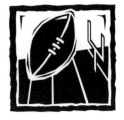

**WHEN I HIRED A TRAINER AT MY GYM,** she completely redesigned my exercise program. She created a weight-training program for me, and she encouraged me to do interval training, keeping my heart rate in the training range. When I moved across the country a few months ago, the first thing I did was find a gym; the second was to hire a new personal trainer. There's an extra cost, but it's absolutely, positively one of the best things I've ever done.

—*LAURA VINCENT*
*SAN RAFAEL, CALIFORNIA*
*LBS. LOST 80*

**ONCE I STARTED WORKING OUT**, I became a lot more health-conscious. You go past McDonald's, and you might have that craving, but I think, "Hey, I just worked out." I was watching everything I put in my body. When I don't work out, I feel guilty.

—*JOE*
*MILWAUKEE, WISCONSIN*
*LBS. LOST 25*

**I LIKE TO THINK** I get my exercise at work every day. I walk around a lot between buildings and offices. By the time I get home I feel like I have run a marathon!

—*ANONYMOUS*
*NEW YORK, NEW YORK*
*LBS. LOST 20*

# Last Resort: The Plus and Minus of Modern Medicine

T his is the 21st century! With all the advances humankind has made over the years, is your only option for losing weight really to deprive yourself of foods you love and exercise until your blisters have blisters? Can't modern medicine offer anything to take the pain—and pounds—away? Obviously, you need to ask your physician, but let's see what some of the people we talked to have to suggest.

I HAVE TRIED EVERY DIET known to mankind. About eight years ago I lost 60 pounds, but in the end, I gained it all back and remained unsuccessful in my weight-loss attempts until I had gastric bypass surgery.

—ANN MOUSNER
MURIETTA, CALIFORNIA
LBS. LOST 118

DIET PILLS ARE WORTHLESS. ENERGY PILLS ARE BETTER.

—STEPHANIE CONE
MONROE, IOWA
LBS. LOST 20

**ALL DIET PILLS HAVE TO BE APPROVED** by the FDA, so if the government says they are safe and your doctor says they are safe, I don't think you have a lot to worry about. I know they worked for me. Nothing else seemed to work because I couldn't stop eating and I didn't have the energy to exercise. As soon as I started with the medication, the weight just melted off.

—*GINA PETRARSKI*
*POLAND, OHIO*
*LBS. LOST 23*

· · · · · · · · ·

## SURGERY STAT

The average weight of individuals who opt for surgery as a cure for obesity is 279.4 pounds.

**PRESCRIPTION DIET PILLS** are very strong drugs, and some of them have dangerous side effects. Be sure to talk to a doctor before taking this route. I was taking diet pills for a while and they were working, but I couldn't sleep at night. I was down to about two hours a night before I went to see the doctor, and he took me off of them. Of course the weight went back on.

—*TODD COOPER*
*YOUNGSTOWN, OHIO*
*LBS. LOST 12*

· · · · · · · · ·

**PEOPLE WHO HAVE GASTRIC BYPASS SURGERY** need to know that it's a life-altering event. When someone goes on a diet, the next day they can decide to throw it out the window and have a chocolate sundae. Not so if you have the surgery. If you overeat, you throw up. If you overeat enough times, your stomach will stretch and defeat the purpose of the surgery. I can only eat a few bites of food at a time, so going out to dinner has been interesting because people are so used to eating huge portions. The waitress will often come up to me and ask, "Was everything OK?"

—*LAURA SIGHINOLFI*
*BOCA RATON, FLORIDA*
*LBS. LOST 150*

# DON'T HOLD YOUR BREATH

A perfect diet pill still does not exist, and none is likely to appear for purchase anytime soon, although there are some new drugs available which are being touted as safer and more effective than the diet pills of the past, some of which included amphetamines, thyroid hormone, fenfluramine, ephedra and phenylpropanolamine. However, these new drugs cannot facilitate weight loss without calorie reduction, will not keep weight off without continued calorie cutting, exercise and use of the drug, and only reduce weight an average of five to ten percent. Although some doctors regard obesity as a chronic disease which must be continually treated, the medication is expensive, and the average weight loss is hardly enough to really help a morbidly obese patient.

The two most popular drugs now on the market are Meridia, which reduces hunger, increases feelings of fullness, and prevents metabolic rate from dropping as a result of weight loss, and Xenical, which acts on the enzyme that digests fat and causes it to be absorbed, cutting fat absorption by a third. Meridia causes weight losses of about 10 to 14 pounds in six months, and Xenical can help patients keep off about 10 percent of their body weight (in a study, one quarter of participants on the drug kept the weight off for four years, while only sixteen percent of those on a placebo did), but fat intake must be limited to 20 grams per day.

# RESIST THE URGE

Walk away from those horrific diet pills! Listen to the pleas of a young woman who has battled weight loss and gain all her life. My immune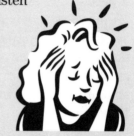
system is shattered from the countless pills I took each day so I could have the slender body of my dreams. When I was taking diet pills I had frequent vomiting and an intense feeling of hunger. I put myself at risk for heart attacks, strokes, and even death.

Diet pills alone will not solve your weight problems. You must do the obvious, such as exercise and eat balanced meals, to lose weight in a healthy way. Speak with a nutritionist. She will formulate a proper diet plan that suits your needs. However, the one element you need to replace those diet pills with is determination. You must have determination within yourself to lose weight and achieve your goal.

—STEPHANIE NOLASCO
NEW YORK, NEW YORK
LBS. LOST 10

**I LOST WEIGHT WITH** gastric bypass surgery. It was amazing—I lost 15 pounds in the first week alone. Like any surgery, it helps to be prepared. I had a tube in my nose for 24 hours after the surgery, which made it hard to talk or swallow. My incision hurt for about a week. But after that I could walk and sit up straight with no problem. For the first two weeks, I ate only broth, Jell-O, and popsicles. For two weeks after that, I could only eat foods that were smooth, such as mashed potatoes. Since then, though, I can eat pretty much anything—just in smaller amounts. So far I've lost more than 100 pounds in eight months, and I've gone from a size 28 to a 12!

—CHRISTINA COLON
NEW YORK, NEW YORK
LBS. LOST 106

Diet pills scare me. If I can't put chocolate and pizza in my mouth, then I'm not putting some drug in me, either!

—J.S.
IOWA CITY, IOWA
LBS. LOST 25

# A NEW SURGICAL SIDE EFFECT

More than 140,000 Americans had surgery to promote weight loss last year; most of them were gastric bypasses. Although the operation is often considered the only solution for many obese people, it may have some unwelcome and dangerous side effects. Lately, doctors have been noticing a rise in cases of patients who, after having undergone bypass surgery, experienced unpredictable and often very severe bouts of hypoglycemia, or drops in blood sugar, one to three hours after eating. With testing, doctors found that the surgery had the side effect of throwing the pancreas into overdrive, producing enormous amounts of insulin. In many cases patients opted to remove more than half of their pancreas in order to keep insulin levels in check.

**BEFORE YOU HAVE GASTRIC BYPASS SURGERY** start eating a lot of protein. After surgery, that will be your focus. Now, I eat nothing that doesn't have some protein in it.

—*MELANIE LUKEN*
*VACAVILLE, CALIFORNIA*
*LBS. LOST 107*

＂Miracle fat-burning pills, machines that exercise for you, and fad diets are all what they seem: too good to be true. There's only one way to lose weight and get in shape: Eat less, eat healthy, and exercise more.＂

—*B.H.*
*SEATTLE, WASHINGTON*

**BEFORE YOU TAKE DIET PILLS**, you have to ask yourself if it's worth it to drop a couple of pounds. It might be easier to just do some sit-ups. Some diet pills, especially the stimulant-based ones, are addictive and can be abused. Abuse then leads to dependence. I got hooked on diet pills before I even realized what was happening.

—*JANET DOMBROUS*
*POLAND, OHIO*
*LBS. LOST 14*

# WEIGHT LOSS WITHOUT DIETING

*Cutting-edge research has yielded some interesting strategies for getting—and staying—slim. Here are a few of the most recent:*

A new study shows that calcium interferes with the hormone that causes fat to be stored. In practice, a 24-week test showed that the group that added three to four servings of low-fat dairy products to their diet lost about nine pounds more per week than the group that did not. However, the test subjects were following a reduced calorie diet as well. Simply adding calcium to your present diet will not bring about weight loss.

In order to produce serotonin, the chemical in the brain that controls our moods, the body requires carbohydrates and sunlight. Therefore, staying inside during the day may cause serotonin levels to fall, increasing your carb cravings. Reduction of serotonin is one reason that people tend to get cranky on low carb diets!

In a study performed at a Cornell University Super Bowl party, snacks were served in bowls of two sizes: gallon and half-gallon. At the end of the evening, those who had served themselves from the gallon bowls had eaten 50 percent more than those who had eaten from the smaller bowls.

The mineral chromium keeps the body's insulin levels down, which may affect weight gain. Overweight test subjects who took chromium for ten years gained around 11 pounds less than those who did not. The study's author recommends a supplement of 200 micrograms daily.

Long-term weight loss can be effected by eating more fruit and not less. After six years, adults who ate more fruit either lost or kept off more weight than those who ate less.

# THE GOOD AND THE BAD

Surgery had a dramatic and positive impact on my health very quickly. Prior to surgery, I took 10 prescription drugs daily (two of them insulin). After six months, I am down to one insulin dose and three pills, and all of these are half of the previous dosages. Before my surgery, I couldn't walk or stand for more than 10 minutes, so I made all my decisions about going out based on how long I would have to walk or stand. I couldn't stoop or bend over, and I couldn't wear shoes because my feet and legs swelled so badly that nothing fit. Now that I've lost the weight, there is little or nothing I can't do.

But surgery had other, less positive effects on my life. Eating out after gastric bypass surgery is a huge challenge. People I go out with sometimes feel uncomfortable if I don't eat along with them, but I enjoy the social aspect of going out. People who have not had the surgery do not always understand this.

The surgery also affected my marriage. Oddly, everyone in my family was very supportive of my decision to have gastric bypass surgery, except my husband. He couldn't stand my weight but was dead-set against the surgery. We ended up separating nine months before I had it. He has since changed his mind about the procedure after seeing how much healthier and happier I am.

—MICHELE WALTON
BUENA PARK, CALIFORNIA
LBS. LOST 107

**AFTER SURGERY MY DOCTOR** advised me not to eat red meat, drink carbonated soda, or take most over-the-counter medications. I rarely drink alcohol. I'm a cheap date now; one drink is fine and if I have two I'll be dancing on the bar. I take 20 vitamins a day and drink a protein shake each day. All of these changes are because of the dramatic overhaul that has been done to my stomach and intestines.

—LAURA SIGHINOLFI
BOCA RATON, FLORIDA
LBS. LOST *150*

• • • • • • • •

## SURGERY STAT

**Five years after gastric-bypass surgery, the average patient is able to keep off 60 percent of his original weight.**

**I FIRST WANTED TO HAVE** the surgery five years ago but didn't pass the psychological evaluation. I was raising my child by myself and didn't have the support to help during the post surgical time. Once that changed, I looked into the procedure again. The gold standard is gastric bypass, but there are other kinds of surgery, such as the duodenal switch, which is for people who need to lose more than 200 pounds, and the Rouen-Y. I learned a lot from *www.obesityhealth.com*, which has information, 24-hour peer support, chat rooms, message boards, and also provides help regarding the insurance approval process.

—MELANIE LUKEN
VACAVILLE, CALIFORNIA
LBS. LOST *107*

• • • • • • • •

**ANY BAD RELATIONSHIPS** you have before surgery will most likely end after surgery. As our confidence grows, we let go of things in our lives that harm us.

—CYNTHIA REYNOLDS
ANAHEIM, CALIFORNIA
LBS. LOST *142*

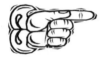

**AFTER GASTRIC BYPASS SURGERY,** I had to relearn how to eat. Now I eat slower and the consistency of my food needs to be moist, otherwise it does not go down well. In the first six months, a piece of food may not go down for a myriad of reasons, and there can be numerous episodes of throwing up. Also, if you are prone to nasal issues, the dripping can also cause you to throw up. But this phase passes with time.

—*CYNTHIA REYNOLDS*
*ANAHEIM, CALIFORNIA*
*LBS. LOST 142*

# Friends and Foes: Family, Diet Partners, and Secret Saboteurs

*A*s you work toward your weight-loss goals, your family and friends can be either your biggest cheerleaders, or your biggest roadblocks. Here's how to get slim with a little help from your friends—or in spite of it.

**GET A DIETING BUDDY** (preferably not your husband, wife, or mother-in-law). Choose a friend who you know will encourage you and pick you up when you fall.

—*LORI B.*
*CHARLESTON, SOUTH CAROLINA*
*LBS. LOST 10*

**DIET WITH A FRIEND. MISERY LOVES COMPANY.**

—*JILL FULLEN*
*PITTSBURGH, PENNSYLVANIA*
*LBS. LOST 13*

## CUT THE CAKE

Mom just isn't making dessert anymore: A recent study found that only 15 percent of dinners made at home include dessert, a decrease of 6 percent since 1990.

**ONE OF THE BEST THINGS** about losing weight is the way it rubs off on your family. As I was losing weight, my husband lost 35 pounds just by eating what I was eating and exercising along with me. Our kids are all into exercise, too. For example, our youngest daughter does weight training and kickboxing, and swims competitively on her high school team. It's great to be such a positive influence on them!

—*Joan Rainwater*
*Waterville, Ohio*
*lbs. lost 37*

• • • • • • • • •

**SURROUND YOURSELF WITH** supportive people. My husband helped me to stay on course, and even when I would get discouraged he kept me focused. He would call me after I left the LA Weight Loss center to see how I did. He would congratulate me if I lost weight or encourage me if I hadn't lost an ounce.

—*Karen Buffum*
*Round Rock, Texas*
*lbs. lost 25*

• • • • • • • • •

**LOSING WEIGHT HAS BENEFITED** my whole family. My husband lost 20 pounds just by eating the foods that I was cooking and eating. Plus, I started buying foods like Healthy Life bread, which is lower in calories than most breads, and my son doesn't know the difference; a peanut butter-and-jelly sandwich tastes just the same on it. At our family events, I used to serve standard picnic fare. But now I offer vegetables and fruit and grilled chicken. When I visit my family, I notice that they are changing what they serve, too. They may still serve hamburgers, but they'll have chicken, too.

—*Karen Phillips*
*Lansing, Illinois*
*lbs. lost 42*

**MY HUSBAND THOUGHT** he was being supportive by giving me a "look" every time I broke my diet. I found myself waiting until he left for work so I could binge in secret. Until I learned how to tell him to back off, I was angry and self-destructive. Tell your well-meaning spouse that you appreciate his or her support, but you need to do this your way.

—SHARI BRADHAM
GREENSBORO, NORTH CAROLINA
LBS. LOST 10

· · · · · · · · ·

"I asked a friend in the office to say, 'Stacy, remember how your arms looked in that dress!' every time I order unhealthy foods. This helps me eat well!"

—STACY
TORONTO, ONTARIO, CANADA

· · · · · · · · ·

**MY HUSBAND WANTED TO LOSE** some weight and I wanted to be healthy as well as support him, so we decided to diet together. It was good for him to have a partner in crime to help him stick to the plan. My husband did really well and was happy with his results after his diet last year. When you see progress it encourages you to keep going.

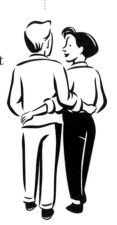

—ANONYMOUS
SONOMA, CALIFORNIA

# WEIGHT AND YOUR CHILDREN

**HAVING LITTLE KIDS AROUND THE HOUSE** while you're dieting is a good thing because they require so much energy on your part that you can't help but lose weight. I even started doing stuff that I would normally ask them to do in order to burn more calories. I still make them help out around the house, but I do more of it myself—especially if it involves going upstairs.

> —MARK TOOMEY
> BOARDMAN, OHIO
> LBS. LOST 6

**WHEN YOU'RE DEALING WITH YOUNG CHILDREN,** try to promote healthy eating in goofy ways. I will say to my four-year-old daughter, "Let me see your muscles," then challenge her to an arm-wrestling match. After she loses, I'll reply, "You'd better eat a piece of broccoli if you want to get stronger." She will eat it and immediately afterward we'll arm wrestle again, and I'll let her win. My response? "See what that broccoli did for you?" For days after, she'll want to eat broccoli all the time to get strong!

> —RANDY FREITIK
> PEORIA, ILLINOIS

**LITTLE KIDS ARE A GOOD BAROMETER** for what foods you can and cannot eat on a diet. They will eat anything that you shouldn't be eating. If I have a Twinkie and ask them to eat it, they will—so I know I shouldn't. If I have some carrots, and the kids say no, then I know it's OK to eat.

> —J.H.
> POLAND, OHIO
> LBS. LOST 13

**WHEN YOU HAVE KIDS AROUND,** keep the junk food in a cabinet that you do not use for everyday cooking. At least that way you don't have to see it every time you need a cup of flour. You're still going to see the stuff when the kids are eating it, but hopefully they eat fast.

—*G.T.*
*YOUNGSTOWN, OHIO*
*LBS. LOST 16*

. . . . . . . . .

**IT'S MY HUSBAND, NOT MY KIDS,** who insists on the sweet cereal at the grocery store.

—*L.G.*
*ATLANTA, GEORGIA*
*LBS. LOST 26*

. . . . . . . .

**I'M PRETTY LAISSEZ-FAIRE ABOUT** what the kids eat, mostly because they exercise of their own accord. They see me do it daily, and I think that has provided an indication to them that this is important.

—*ANDREA COX*
*GRAND LAKE, COLORADO*
*LBS. LOST 30*

. . . . . . . .

**TO GET KIDS INVOLVED, MAKE EXERCISE FUN.** I like to exercise to old Richard Simmons tapes. Sometimes my teenage daughters join in, too. We used to do this when they were little, so I think they get a kick out of it.

—*MOLLY BROWN*
*ALLENTOWN, PENNSYLVANIA*

# PATHS TO GOOD HABITS

*Many experts and advisors, including television talk show host Dr. Phil, recommend applying brainpower when beginning a weight-loss program. It's a major project, and you should approach it like a project manager or an Army officer; in other words, get organized!*

- Have a definite goal in mind when you start your diet. Ask yourself how many pounds you want to lose, and imagine yourself at that weight to keep yourself on track.

- You're not going to lose any weight just by thinking about it—you need a planned approach that includes dieting and exercise.

- Consider giving a friend or relative progress reports—if you know you're going to have to 'fess up later, you'll be more likely to stay focused. In addition, their support will help you through your failures *and* your successes.

- Approach your diet in increments, with small and manageable steps that are right for *your* life. But make sure that these steps are leading towards a positive life goal, not just being less fat.

- Put your weight-loss goals on a timeline that's both realistic and inspiring. Try to think of what you'd like to achieve in one year, and fit your smaller goals to the timeline.

**I'M VERY LUCKY TO HAVE SUPPORTIVE** coworkers. They all eat very healthy, and they have been very encouraging to me. In the past, I didn't eat any vegetables at all, but my coworkers encouraged me to try a new vegetable every week. Now I enjoy carrots, tomatoes, and even celery. I just made a batch of chicken noodle soup with both carrots and celery in it!

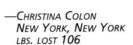

> —CHRISTINA COLON
> NEW YORK, NEW YORK
> LBS. LOST *106*

* * * * * * *

**I SAY THAT WHEN YOU ARE ON A DIET** nobody in the house is allowed to eat anything that you can't eat. It has to be a team effort. If they complain too much, tell them the quicker they help you lose the weight, the quicker they can have their candy bars back.

> —CHARLOTTE KUBALY
> POLAND, OHIO
> LBS. LOST *8*

* * * * * * *

**SEEK OUT SUPPORT WHEREVER** you can get it. It makes a big difference. When my kids say, "Mom, you're doing great!" it gives me such a boost.

> —RHODA
> PROVO, UTAH
> LBS. LOST *45*

# EQUAL OPPORTUNITY

As children, boys are more likely to be overweight than girls (33 percent versus 28 percent). By the time they reach their teens, however, the scales are balanced (so to speak), and both males and females have a 30 percent chance of being overweight.

# EATING OVERTIME: OFFICE LEFTOVERS

Having a partner at work helps sustain your diet. At my work, they do a lot of catered food for meetings, and there's always leftover food in our work area, like cookies, cinnamon rolls and stuffed pizza. It's such good food that even after eating your own lunch it's hard to pass up eating some of this food. My coworker and I were struggling with this. We knew we shouldn't be eating junk, but it was hard to pass up. I came up with this idea: We have a pact where we are allowed to splurge once a week, but the rest of the time we pass it up. We went cold turkey, and found it's been much easier to control what we're eating when we know 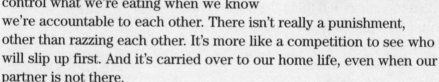 we're accountable to each other. There isn't really a punishment, other than razzing each other. It's more like a competition to see who will slip up first. And it's carried over to our home life, even when our partner is not there.

—WADE
AURORA, ILLINOIS
LBS. LOST 10

**MY HUSBAND WANTED ME** to drop a few pounds, but he had the good sense not to come right out and say it. If he had done that he would have been sleeping in the dog house for a while. But he has been supportive, and that is so important. The nicest thing he does for me is to eat his meatball sandwiches at work. He knows how I lust for those.

—*MITZIE HAGEN*
*WHEELING, WEST VIRGINIA*
*LBS. LOST 16*

- - - - - - - -

**DON'T BE AFRAID TO TELL FRIENDS,** relatives and even your coworkers about your diet. A lot of us are sheepish about dieting. If you're honest, you'll find that lots of people share your struggles and frustrations. You'll have people to celebrate with when you reach a weight-loss goal. You'll be less likely to reach for a Twinkie if you know your friends are pulling for you to succeed. And if you do eat that Twinkie, you can confess to your friends, instead of letting guilt consume you.

—*ANNA DUBROVSKY*
*SANTA MONICA, CALIFORNIA*

- - - - - - - -

**NEVER, UNDER ANY CIRCUMSTANCES,** make a negative, weight-related comment to your wife. When my wife was pregnant, I made the mistake of asking her if pregnancy made you gain weight all over, because it looked like that was happening to her. She was extremely upset for a week, to the point where she even cried about it. I felt horrible. She's tried many diets throughout the years, and no matter how well they do or don't work, the only comments that come out of my mouth are things like, "You have great curves," or "You carry yourself well."

—*RANDY FREITIK*
*PEORIA, ILLINOIS*

**HOLIDAY GAME PLAN**

To fight weight gain over the holidays, combine gatherings with physical activity, such as touch football or a walk around the neighborhood.

**BEING PART OF A WEIGHT-LOSS** support group at work has been very helpful to me; if I try to lose the weight by myself it might not work. We're like a big family. We exchange stories and recipes, and each week we report how much weight we lost. This is very powerful for me because I love to eat, but the thought that I'll have to report to the group often keeps me from eating something unhealthy.

—*LORETTA*
   *OREM, UTAH*
   LBS. LOST *15*

· · · · · · · ·

" As a Christmas gift, one of my daughters gave me a low-fat cookbook, which turned out to be very useful. I enjoyed preparing low-fat meals that also tasted good. "

—*MICHAEL BYRNE*
   *GIBBSTOWN, NEW JERSEY*
   LBS. LOST *20*

· · · · · · · ·

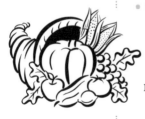

**MY KIDS EAT MORE VEGETABLES NOW:** I'd never really offered them before. The first time my four-year-old asked for another carrot I nearly cried, I was so happy.

—*KAREN PHILLIPS*
   *LANSING, ILLINOIS*
   LBS. LOST *42*

# THE POWER OF FRIENDS AND FAMILY

My husband has been amazing. He never complained about any of the changes I made in my cooking, the snacks that disappeared from our cabinets, the hours I initially spent in the grocery store aisles reading all the labels. He lost 40 pounds just because of the changes I made in my cooking and by staying out of fast-food places.

My mom stocks the foods I can eat and has changed a lot of her cooking habits so that when my husband and I go over there to eat, it is healthy. She has been my number one cheerleader.

My best friend, who has never had a weight problem, celebrated every single ounce I lost with me. When I hit the "100 pounds lost" mark, she and another one of my closest friends sent me a huge basket of 100 yellow and white daisies (which happen to be my favorite flower).

The person who gave me the most incentive was my father. I watched him, at 64 years old, lose a leg and lose a portion of his other foot a year later, and never slow down. He has a prosthesis, and he has never been through a moment's therapy, yet he does everything he wants to do including fishing, hunting (yes, he climbs trees), and driving. I realized that somewhere I had that same willpower; I just had to find it.

Although I take the credit for losing the weight, I give all these the people the recognition they deserve for standing beside me and holding my hand and loving me, no matter what.

—KANDI KIZZIAH
ROCKY MOUNT, NORTH CAROLINA
LBS. LOST 158

**FAT STAT**

Obesity in adults has a direct effect on children. Overweight children aged 10 to 14 with at least one obese parent have a 79 percent chance of being overweight as adults.

**JOINING A WEIGHT-LOSS SUPPORT GROUP** really helps. When I tell my husband that I've lost a pound he says, "Great." But when I tell the members of my weight-loss group, I get a round of applause! If one of us discovers a new healthy salad dressing, she'll bring it in for us all to taste. We even bring guest speakers into our meetings to learn more about weight loss. So far we've had a yoga instructor and a college professor speak.

—DAPHNE
OREM, UTAH
LBS. LOST 47

• • • • • • • • •

**TRY TO DIET WITH YOUR SPOUSE,** partner, or roommate. When there are two of you, it's easier to portion the food, choose what to eat, and control what comes in the house. Also, try to have lots of stuff in the refrigerator that you can eat. When you open the refrigerator door, you're often confronted by stuff you want and can't have. Try to pack the house with things you can have—like cheese sticks, fruit, diet soda, etc.

—DEBBIE SMITH
NEW YORK, NEW YORK

• • • • • • • • •

**IT'S WONDERFUL IF YOU HAVE** support during your weight loss, but it's just as great, if not better, to encourage other people. I was so pleased with the NutriSystem program that 13 of my friends and family also joined! It was not a difficult task to convince them, since they were already impressed by my results. My aunt has struggled with her weight since I can remember, and witnessing her lose 26 pounds on the program was a joy for me.

—ZORA ANDRICH
LAMBERTVILLE, NEW JERSEY
LBS. LOST 20

# ONE THING YOUR SPOUSE SHOULD NEVER SAY

**THEY SHOULD NEVER SAY** that you are going to die if you don't lose some weight. I don't think negative comments should ever be used as motivation. And death is the ultimate negative.

> —*TOM RHODES*
> *CAMPBELL, OHIO*
> *LBS. LOST 5*

**WORDING IS CRITICAL.** I asked my wife how she thought my diet was going, and she said, "You're not as fat as you were." I'm sure she meant to say that I looked like I had lost some weight.

> —*E.P.*
> *CRANBERRY TOWNSHIP, PENNSYLVANIA*
> *LBS. LOST 14*

**THEY SHOULD NOT SAY ANYTHING AT ALL.** It's not like I'm blind. I can see that I'm fat, I don't need to hear it from her.

> —*CARL PALONE*
> *BOARDMAN, OHIO*
> *LBS. LOST 7*

**EVEN SUGGESTIONS CAN SOUND LIKE CRITICISM** to someone on a diet. It's presumptuous for my husband to tell me not to eat some potato chips if I am having a craving. I tell him it's better that I have a few chips now than to eat the whole bag and kill the whole diet.

> —*T.M.*
> *PITTSBURGH, PENNSYLVANIA*
> *LBS. LOST 12*

**MY WIFE ALWAYS TELLS ME THAT** I'm not as fat as my brother—he weighs 350 pounds! I know she's just trying to help, but she's failing.

> —*RAY BALLAST*
> *BOARDMAN, OHIO*
> *LBS. LOST 8*

**DON'T TEMPT YOUR PARTNER** if she is dieting. If she is sitting there watching TV, and you get out a bag of potato chips and start eating in front of her, that's not very nice. I've tempted my wife and daughter many times. It takes a certain amount of self-control on my part not to.

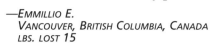

—*EMMILLIO E.*
*VANCOUVER, BRITISH COLUMBIA, CANADA*
*LBS. LOST 15*

* * * * * * * *

" The changes that people make to improve the way they cook and eat will help their families, too. Because I changed how I cook, my 15-year-old daughter lost eight pounds, and my husband lost 10 pounds. "

—*DIANE SZYMANSKI*
*SOUTH BEND, INDIANA*
*LBS. LOST 72*

* * * * * * * *

**DON'T CONSTANTLY COMPARE YOURSELF** to your friends because the diet that works for them may not suit your lifestyle.

—*JEFFREY TOCKMAN*
*SAN FRANCISCO, CALIFORNIA*
*LBS. LOST 15*

**EVERYONE IN MY LIFE** has been extremely support-ive, cheering me every inch of the way. There were weeks, of course, when the scale stayed the same. That is when they were all most vocal with support. My husband and children were my biggest cheerleaders: They knew I could accom-plish this before I did.

—*PATRICIA MICHENER*
*WEST GROVE, PENNSYLVANIA*
*LBS. LOST 146*

**FAT STAT**

About 15 percent of all children and teens in the United States are over-weight, more than double the percent-age in the early 1970s.

**MY SPOUSE HAS NEVER UTTERED** a negative word about my appearance before, during, or after a diet. He constantly says that I am beautiful and that as long as I feel healthy and happy, he's happy. He has offered to exercise with me as well. We go on walks and hikes, and he swims with me.

—*ANONYMOUS*
*BIRMINGHAM, ALABAMA*
*LBS. LOST 30*

**STAY AWAY FROM YOUR HUSBAND'S VEHICLE** when you're dieting. While I was doing Weight Watchers, my husband would hoard cookies and chocolate in his truck so I wouldn't find them. This was the ideal hiding place because I would never go anywhere near his truck.

—*S.A.*
*LAKE FOREST, CALIFORNIA*
*LBS. LOST 15*

**AVOID EVERYONE WITH WHOM** you enjoy eating and drinking.

—*A.M.*
*CAMBRIDGE, MASSACHUSETTS*

**DIET ETIQUETTE**

What to say to Grandma when she offers you a fattening dessert at her house: "It looks so good, but I am so full."

**I** JOINED **WEIGHT WATCHERS** with another mother from my daughter's school who wasn't even a close friend, but she's been a tremendous help, and we've become good buddies. We've gone through the thick together; hopefully we'll get to the thin soon!

—*Lori B.*
*Charleston, South Carolina*
*lbs. lost 10*

# Out of Your Element: Taking Your Diet on the Road

I t's one thing to stick to your diet when you're at home, presumably in control of stocking the fridge and cooking for yourself. But it's a challenge to maintain healthy eating habits when you're away from home—at a restaurant, a party, or on a trip. Here's how to take your weight-loss show on the road.

**EATING OUT WHILE DIETING IS FRUSTRATING,** especially when you are with friends who can eat their body weight in cheese and chocolate without gaining an ounce.

—*CHRISTINE WARREN*
*RAINBOW CITY, ALABAMA*
*LBS. LOST 30*

**IF YOU GO OUT TO A RESTAURANT, EAT HALF OF WHAT YOU'RE SERVED.**

—*BRONLEA HAWKINS*
*NEW YORK,*
*NEW YORK*

**WHEN I'M TRAVELING**, I make a conscious effort to replace a few of the courses at restaurants with veggies and fruit. I either order salad and soup or ask for a plate of cooked vegetables. It's easy to find this stuff no matter where you go. These days, most restaurants are quite accommodating.

—*EMMILLIO E.*
*VANCOUVER, BRITISH COLUMBIA, CANADA*
*LBS. LOST 15*

* * * * * * * *

" If I have a really strong craving for something sweet, I order a slice of pie or cake at a restaurant rather than making something at home. Then I only get one slice instead of eating the whole cake. "

—*AMY*
*ALBURTIS, PENNSYLVANIA*

* * * * * * * *

**DON'T EAT THE BREAD THEY PUT OUT!** If you have to eat it, have one piece and ask the server to take the basket away immediately. Leaving it on the table is asking for trouble.

—*S.F.*
*BUFFALO GROVE, ILLINOIS*
*LBS. LOST 15*

# IMPROVISE

**I GO CRAZY WHEN I'M SOMEWHERE** where there's no gym. I've figured out how to keep up my exercise schedule while I'm away, though: I walk everywhere, I take the stairs, I do gym exercises with furniture, I lift chairs until it burns. Even if the furniture is light, it's worth doing while you're watching TV in the hotel room. On a recent trip I did curls with my baby nephew!

> —PETER STEUR
> BRISBANE, AUSTRALIA
> LBS. LOST 25

• • • • • • • • •

**FIGURE OUT HOW TO MAKE YOUR SITUATION** work for you. I'm a truck driver, and sometimes I sit for 11 hours straight, which makes it hard to work out. To remedy this, I keep a jump rope and a set of dumbbells in my truck. About three times a week, I do a 30-minute workout at rest stops. I'll jump rope for 15 minutes, then do curls, triceps extensions, and flies with the dumbbells.

> —LENNARD HAYNES SR.
> HOUSTON, TEXAS
> LBS. LOST 40

• • • • • • • • •

**WITH SO MANY HOTELS** having spas and weight rooms, it's possible to get some exercise when you're on a business trip. I usually get more active when I am gone. If I have the time, I walk on the beaches and to restaurants.

> —KIM JAFFE
> REDMOND, WASHINGTON

## NO HOME COOKING

The average American takes out food from restaurants 117 times a year.

I ask my server not to bring the bread basket. That way, I'm not even tempted to indulge.

—*L.A.*
*CLEVELAND, OHIO*
*LBS. LOST 8*

**WHEN YOU GO OUT TO EAT,** if you don't see something on the menu that fits into your eating plan, just ask. More likely than not, they'll go out of their way to help you out. Once I was at an ESPN Zone restaurant and I didn't see a thing on the menu that I could eat. So, I asked the waiter if they had any fruit. He brought me out a fresh apple. It was perfect!

—*DIANE SZYMANSKI*
*SOUTH BEND, INDIANA*
*LBS. LOST 72*

• • • • • • • • •

**MOST OF US CAN BE GOOD** little boys and girls when we're at home with our cupboards that have been cleansed of all bad stuff. At home is also where we keep our little scale to measure our portions just so. But when we're out among the beautiful people under the lights of a nice restaurant—well, that's when temptation often gets the best of us. I always think to myself, "Is that half-pound cheeseburger with all the fattening trimmings, and with the seasoned-cut French fries on the side, really worth throwing away a week's worth of hard work for?" The answer is always no, but it's still tough.

—*DYLAN TOOMEY*
*WHEELING, WEST VIRGINIA*

• • • • • • • • •

**IF I HAD IT MY WAY,** I'd eat Italian every night. But when you go to that kind of restaurant it seems that every piece of food is filled with carbs and cheese. I let myself eat as much bread, oil, and Parmesan cheese as I want, but I order a healthier main course like grilled shrimp, or pasta and tomato sauce.

—*BUZZ ORR*
*EVANSTON, ILLINOIS*
*LBS. LOST 15*

I LIVE IN NEW YORK CITY, home of diverse cuisines. I love eating out. For me, Japanese restaurants and sushi bars offer great options. Indian restaurants are also good, especially the tandoori and veggie dishes. I also love salad bars, and places where good salads are part of the menu. Just remember, you are the customer. Do not be afraid to ask the questions that will support you.

—*DEB WUNDER*
*BROOKLYN, NEW YORK*
*LBS. LOST 36*

**RISKY BEHAVIOR**
Those who eat fast food twice a week for 15 years are an average of 10 pounds heavier, and have twice the risk of developing type-2 diabetes than those who eat fast food less than once a week.

I EAT OUT A LOT AND HAVE TO MAKE a real effort to stop eating when I'm full. I know that if the plate sits in front of me, I'll keep picking at the food, so I ask the waiter to take my plate right away. If that's not possible, I'll pour salt over everything or even put my napkin on the plate (not classy, but it works).

—*LHASA MANOR*
*PHILADELPHIA, PENNSYLVANIA*
*LBS. LOST 45*

I BRING MY LUNCH to work so I can control what I'm eating and how much.

—*MICHELE HENRY*
*TORONTO, ONTARIO, CANADA*
*LBS. LOST 5*

# DON'T ASK, DON'T TELL

By law, restaurants are not required to provide nutrition information for a menu item unless a nutrient-content claim (such as low fat, fat free, reduced fat) or a health claim (such as "diets low in saturated fat, trans fat and cholesterol may reduce the risk of heart disease") is made.

# LET THE GOOD TIMES ROLL

**NEVER TRY TO DIET ON VACATION.** You won't enjoy yourself if you're constantly worrying about food. I was on Atkins and spent a week in Mexico. I tried for a day to stay on it, but I was miserable. When you're sitting on the beach, you want a sugary drink. At night, you want bread with your dinner: It's just that simple. You're on vacation, so let it go.

> —*ABBY*
> *CHICAGO, ILLINOIS*
> *LBS. LOST 20*

* * * * * * * * *

**I CAN'T BELIEVE PEOPLE WORRY** about dieting when they're on vacation. That defeats the whole mindset of enjoying yourself and getting away from the things you normally do. When I'm on vacation, I don't do formal workouts, and I usually have dessert. When I get home, however, the first thing I do is step on the scale and see how much vacation I've had.

> —*DEBBIE REDDEN-BRUNELLO*
> *TEMECULA, CALIFORNIA*
> *LBS. LOST 30*

* * * * * * * * *

**ON VACATIONS, YOU HAVE TO EAT!** If I'm visiting San Francisco and I want to try some of the delicious seafood that city is known for, guess what? I'm going to have it. And, if I'm gone for a week and I come home and find out I've gained two pounds, so what? Once you return to your normal routine, the pounds will come off. But the memories you made will last a lifetime.

> —*P.O.*
> *NEW BRUNSWICK, NEW JERSEY*
> *LBS. LOST 50*

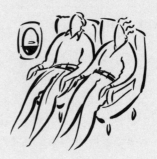

**IF I KNOW I'M GOING OUT** to a restaurant I usually scale back on eating during the day. I don't starve myself, I just limit snacks, or eat fewer carbs and fats. At the restaurant, I limit myself to one piece of bread (if it's on the table) and one glass of wine. And, if the meal portion is huge, I won't eat it all. I'll ask for them to box half of it up so I can take it home with me.

—*MARGARET STECK*
*SEATTLE, WASHINGTON*
LBS. LOST *38*

## RISKY BEHAVIOR #2

When dining out, people clean their plates 67 percent of the time.

**SOME RESTAURANTS JUST MAKE** it harder on you: At California Pizza Kitchen they give you a basket of bread when most everyone in the place is ordering a pizza! It's as if they are trying to help you pig out.

—*ABBY*
*CHICAGO, ILLINOIS*
LBS. LOST *20*

**DON'T GO TO THE PARTY HUNGRY.** Eat a mini-meal first.

—*NAN GEER*
*JACKSONVILLE, FLORIDA*
LBS. LOST *15*

# MORE EVERYTHING

America may be the land of the free, but it's also the home of the super size. One study found that a large order of French fries in the United Kingdom contained 446 calories. But on our side of the pond, a large order of fries has a third more—610 calories.

**CHOOSE A DISH THAT'S GRILLED OR BAKED.** Instead of getting fries, order a baked potato or an extra veggie. Avoid eating too much bread, and instead of alcohol order a diet soda and water with a slice of lemon. If you do this, you won't feel like you cheated on your diet and you will feel better about socializing during your diet.

—ANONYMOUS
BIRMINGHAM, ALABAMA
LBS. LOST 30

• • • • • • • • •

**EATING IS SUCH A SOCIAL THING** in America. I try to really focus more on the friendship than the food. If you eat bite after bite, letting food be the focus, you really cheat yourself in a lot of ways. If you focus more on the company, then the food is just an added bonus. We are fed by so many more things in life than just food. My girlfriends and I made a pact—we see who can eat the slowest. You're paying for the ambience; You're paying for the service. You should enjoy it for as long as possible.

—DOMINIQUE FARRAR
PETALUMA, CALIFORNIA
LBS. LOST 30

# BIGGER, BUT NOT BETTER

Portion sizes have been growing over the years—and so have calories:

|  | 20 years ago | Today |
|---|---|---|
| French Fries | 210 calories | 610 calories |
| Cheeseburger | 333 calories | 590 calories |
| Two slices of pepperoni pizza | 500 calories | 850 calories |
| A portion of spaghetti and meatballs | 500 calories | 1,025 calories |

**ALWAYS ORDER FROM THE LIGHT MENU,** if it is available. If not, treat yourself to the biggest, most expensive salad on the menu. Salad dressing? Go for it. You've got to feel like you're being just a bit naughty once in awhile. If you don't, you won't maintain your new eating habits and will ultimately fall right back into the old fat trap.

> —JACQUIE MCTAGGART
> INDEPENDENCE, IOWA
> LBS. LOST 45

* * * * * * * *

**SPECIAL OCCASIONS AREN'T SPECIAL** occasions when all you can eat is low-fat, low-carb foods, and vegetables. Birthdays, anniversaries, and vacations are inherently more fun when you're with people you love, and are eating or cooking good food. Food is what brings people together. Fun times weren't made for tofu, bean sprouts, and spray butter. For holidays or any other special occasion, break out the sugar, butter, cheese, potatoes and cakes, and deal with it.

> —A. ORR
> CHICAGO, ILLINOIS
> LBS. LOST 10

* * * * * * * *

**ASK FOR THE NUTRITION BROCHURE** in your favorite fast-food restaurant. If you steer clear of the lethal 600-calorie fries, there are actually some good choices.

> —EVELYN RICHARDS
> SUMMERVILLE, SOUTH CAROLINA
> LBS. LOST 65

**DINING AWAY**

The average American eats out 83 times a year, down from a decade ago, when the number was 95 times a year.

# EATING OUT

Americans consume an estimated 40 percent of their calories outside the home.

## TRAVEL ADVISORY

The healthiest U.S. airport to eat in is Miami: 85 percent of its restaurants offer healthy choices.

**IT'S SO MUCH EASIER TO STAY** on a diet when away from home than when left to my own devices at home. Restaurants are terrific today in that regard. I usually start with a salad with dressing on the side, so I can monitor how much I use. I order extra vegetables, I avoid the bread, and if someone else orders dessert, I order fresh fruit.

—SHARON LONDON
SAN FRANCISCO, CALIFORNIA
LBS. LOST 18

• • • • • • • • •

**IF SOMEONE ELSE BUYS THE FOOD** (i.e., I'm invited to a party or out to dinner), I'll eat anything without guilt, and the calories don't count. The rest of the time, I'm very careful about what I put in my mouth. This is how I manage my splurges. Fortunately, this system works for me because I'm so busy taking care of my children that I only go out once or twice a month.

—JULIE MARTIN SUNICH
TAMPA, FLORIDA
LBS. LOST 53

# Read This: Simple, Everyday, Dieting Tips

*When it comes down to it, the weight-loss war is won or lost on a day-to-day basis. There are only so many holidays and special occasions to contend with, so what you eat each day for breakfast, lunch, and dinner—and all those stolen moments in between—is what really matters. Here are some home-baked tips and strategies to help contend with those daily diet challenges.*

**BE PREPARED FOR HUNGER TO STRIKE!** I always bring snacks like granola bars and carrots. This way, if I'm out of the house and get hungry, I won't be tempted to buy junk food at a drive-through or vending machine.

—*DEANNA*
*MACUNGIE, PENNSYLVANIA*

**DRINK LOTS OF WATER; IT TAKES UP VALUABLE REAL ESTATE IN YOUR STOMACH.**

—*STEPHEN MACKAY*
*SAN FRANCISCO, CALIFORNIA*
*LBS. LOST 10*

**THE HARDEST PART ABOUT DIETING** was learning to slow down when I ate so I had time to realize when I was full! Try to pause, take a breath, and wait a minute or two before taking the next bite.

—*GRACE*
*CHAPEL HILL, NORTH CAROLINA*
*LBS. LOST 5*

" Pick one place at home and one place at work to do all your eating. Be sure you are seated; never eat standing up because then you tend to rush through it. Don't eat anywhere but in that place. It really makes a difference. "

—*C.S.*
*EVANS CITY, PENNSYLVANIA*
*LBS. LOST 18*

**BUY THE FOODS THAT YOU LOVE** and measure them out into healthy portions. For example, I buy a big chocolate bar, break it apart into servings, and place each one in a sandwich bag. That way, I can just get one bag from the cabinet, enjoy that amount, and stop eating.

—*JOAN RAINWATER*
*WATERVILLE, OHIO*
*LBS. LOST 37*

**I'M A NERVOUS, COMPULSIVE EATER,** so the thing that helped me the most was chewing gum. When I'd sit at my desk at work, I'd pop a stick of gum into my mouth instead of snacking. It kept my mouth going, and I found that I snacked less.

—DAVID FEDER
DES MOINES, IOWA
LBS. LOST 6

* * * * * * * *

**IF FAT-FREE SALAD DRESSINGS** do not appeal to you, simply mix your favorite regular dressing with a drop of water or touch of vinegar. You'll use less dressing and have the full flavor you love, but with fewer calories.

—SUSIE GALVEZ
RICHMOND, VIRGINIA
LBS. LOST 121

* * * * * * * *

**CHEW LOTS AND LOTS OF GUM.** You still get the taste and your jaws are still working so part of your brain is confused into thinking that you're eating. I went through pack after pack of Juicy Fruit.

—JOHN STANLEY
EAST PALESTINE, OHIO
LBS. LOST 25

* * * * * * * *

**EVERY SUNDAY,** I spend about an hour cutting up a week's worth of fruits and vegetables and putting them in little baggies. This saves us time, because we can just open the refrigerator and get what we need. It also prevents us from eating too much, because each bag contains a single serving. If I sat down with a bag of chips or pretzels at work, I'd probably go through the whole thing out of boredom.

—JAYME
O'FALLON, MISSOURI

I only eat in the dining room. In front of the television, you are likely to see a commercial for Burger King or Oreos, and you don't need that.

—C.S.
EVANS CITY,
PENNSYLVANIA
LBS. LOST 18

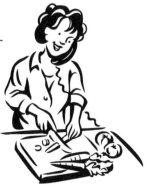

## SLOW AND STEADY

To reach your ideal weight and maintain it, experts recommend a slow and steady weight loss of about 3/4 to 2 pounds per week.

Eat everything with chopsticks. You burn calories and it forces you to eat smaller amounts at a time.

—*N.L.*
*CHICAGO, ILLINOIS*
*LBS. LOST 10*

**I HAVE FIVE WORDS FOR YOU:** Back away from the buffet! All-you-can-eat buffets are the bane of all diets. I avoid them as much as possible. I've found that I eat far too much there, partly out of a need to feel like I've gotten my money's worth and partly out of a desire to try some of everything.

—*ANONYMOUS*
*HELLERTOWN, PENNSYLVANIA*
*LBS. LOST 13*

**ALLOW YOURSELF ONE BAD MEAL** per week. Otherwise, you will go crazy and quit the diet. For me that bad meal meant a breakfast at Burger King. It got me through all that bran cereal I ate for breakfast the rest of the week.

—*RACHEL COSSMAN*
*SOUTH BEND, INDIANA*
*LBS. LOST 110*

**DRINK AS MUCH WATER** as your stomach can hold right before bed. Your body will think you're full and will keep your system running even while you sleep. I lost 60 pounds this way with exercise about twice a week. In addition, you will have a built-in alarm clock when nature calls in the morning.

—*JAMES BOSQUEZ*
*SAN ANTONIO, TEXAS*
*LBS. LOST 60*

**EVEN THOUGH YOU'RE EATING HEALTHY,** don't deny yourself things you crave, or you'll only crave them more. Just eat them in moderation. If you can't live without ice cream, have some. Just don't polish off a pint of Ben & Jerry's and then wonder why your pants are getting tighter.

—*BOB HOLDEN*
*NEW YORK, NEW YORK*

# MULTI-TASK EATING

Everyone knows you're supposed to eat slowly since it takes 20 minutes for your brain to realize you're really full. I've been told to put my fork down between bites or chew each mouthful of food 15 times. That's pretty lame advice as far I'm concerned. You can't exactly put your fork down when you're cleaning the leftover chicken from your kids' plates or straightening out the pie. And who's going to count the times your jaw goes up and down when you're trying to answer the phone, serve dinner, and clean up the grape juice that just spilled?

My advice (which I learned from a dietitian): I pop a piece of sugarless candy in my mouth when I'm getting dinner ready. That way, the clock starts ticking on the 20 minutes before I get to the table. I never get to sit down for 20 minutes anyway, so this way I feel full much faster and eat less.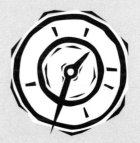

—*Lori B.*
*Charleston, South Carolina*
*lbs. lost 10*

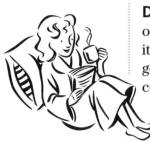

**DRINK COFFEE BEFORE BREAKFAST.** I always have one cup of coffee a day, in the mornings, because it fills me up and gives me more energy, and it gets my metabolism going. When I don't have my coffee, I tend to eat a lot more.

—ANONYMOUS
NEW YORK, NEW YORK
LBS. LOST 25

" I take all the diet magazines I have bought, stack them up, and do step aerobics on them! Seriously, I am a sucker for all of those publications, even though they all say the same thing: Move your butt and don't eat. "

—VELMA WILLARD
BOERNE, TEXAS

**I DON'T EVER WEIGH MYSELF,** except at a doctor's office. I don't really care what the numbers say; what matters is what you look and feel like. Weighing yourself is an easy way to become obsessed. It might be important if you have to lose 50 pounds, but to maintain a healthy lifestyle? That's ridiculous.

—JAYME
O'FALLON, MISSOURI

**BUY BOTTLED WATER.** I know it's more expensive than tap water, but bottled water is more convenient and tastes better than tap. The more water I drink, the easier my weight loss is. In fact, even if I have a day where I indulge, as long as I drink my water the extra food doesn't have as much of an effect. I make sure to take a bottle of water to the gym, drink it while I'm working out, and refill it to drink on the way home.

—*CAROL*
*EASTON, PENNSYLVANIA*
*LBS. LOST* **40**

• • • • • • • •

**SWITCH TO DIET SOFT DRINKS.** I know it sounds like a no-brainer, but some people don't realize how much sugar is in Coke or Pepsi. An average 12-ounce can of regular soda contains around 120 calories, while the diet version usually has one or zero. If you drink three cans a day, you'll be saving 360 calories right there. Multiply that by seven days a week, 30 days a month and 365 days a year. You'll be saving a lot of calories, and that really counts.

—*REILLY BURTON*
*SWISSVALE, PENNSYLVANIA*
*LBS. LOST* **15**

• • • • • • • •

**MAKE SURE TO WEIGH YOURSELF** at a prescribed time every day or every week. But do it under the same conditions. Don't weigh yourself right after breakfast one day and right before bed the next; you will be comparing apples to oranges. I made it a point to weigh myself each day right after I stepped out of the shower. That way I knew the numbers were comparable to the previous day, even if they weren't always encouraging.

—*ANONYMOUS*
*EAST PALESTINE, OHIO*
*LBS. LOST* **7**

## HAPPY EATERS

According to the USDA, most of us are what's known as food optimists—we believe our diets are better than they actually are.

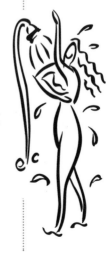

# INSTANT WEIGHT LOSS

**WEARING A BODY-FITTING SHIRT**—preferably dark—underneath something loose, like a blouse or a blazer that covers the hips, gives the illusion of a slimmer frame.

> —*SHERYL LEVINE*
> *NEW YORK, NEW YORK*

. . . . . . . . .

**GET A TAN!**

> —*M.B.*
> *WEEHAWKEN, NEW JERSEY*

. . . . . . . . .

**STAY AWAY FROM SLOPPY CLOTHES.** Think like you're thin and you'll start acting like you're thin.

> —*VI HOWG*
> *MINNETONKA, MINNESOTA*
> *LBS. LOST 26*

. . . . . . . . .

**EVERYONE SHOULD HAVE AN AWESOME,** fitted pair of jeans that look great on you. Invest the money.

> —*ELIZABETH*
> *FORT WAYNE, INDIANA*
> *LBS. LOST 10*

. . . . . . . . .

**THE QUICKEST WAY TO LOOK THIN** is to find some fat friends.

> —*J.A.*
> *IOWA CITY, IOWA*
> *LBS. LOST 15*

. . . . . . . . .

**I WEAR FABULOUS SHOES** because it gives me confidence. If you have that, who cares if you are a size 12 instead of a 2?

> —*PATRICIA*
> *COZUMEL, MEXICO*
> *LBS. LOST 15*

**USE MUSTARD ON YOUR SANDWICHES** instead of mayonnaise. Mustard has no fat and very few calories while mayo is loaded with fat. If you just don't like the taste of mustard, find a low-fat alternative, but avoid mayonnaise at all costs.

—AUDRY WISNESKI
SEWICKLEY, PENNSYLVANIA
LBS. LOST 10

**WHEN A RECIPE CALLS FOR CHEESE,** you can reduce the required amount by using intensely flavored cheeses such as parmesan, gorgonzola, and even sharp, white cheddar. These cheeses are packed with flavor, so less is needed.

—SUSIE GALVEZ
RICHMOND, VIRGINIA
LBS. LOST 121

**YOU SHOULD ALWAYS** have a variety of "friendly" food available, so that if you do feel hungry and really need to eat, you won't be spoiling all your hard work. Friendly foods to keep around: apples, plenty of fresh vegetables, frozen vegetables, fat-free yogurts, fat-free cheese, low-calorie bread and crackers, a pot of thick homemade vegetable soup.

—MIRI GREIDI
RA'ANANA, ISRAEL
LBS. LOST 53

**GET LOTS OF MIRRORS IN YOUR HOME.** Take a good look at yourself. Is it really worth it to keep eating the way you do? Fat people tend to avoid mirrors and scales, but if you take a good look at yourself you won't be able to deny that you need to change your lifestyle.

—BETTY ZAYCHICK
CUMBERLAND, MARYLAND
LBS. LOST 16

I portion out foods that I like—such as sugar-free Jell-O and cottage cheese—into single-serving-size plastic containers. They're easy to grab and go.

—CAROL
EASTON,
PENNSYLVANIA
LBS. LOST 40

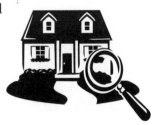

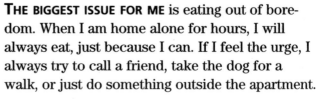

**Doing the paperwork—keeping a food journal, writing down menu plans for the week, preparing shopping lists—is a pain, but it works.**

—*NANCY MCBRIDE*
*NEW ORLEANS,*
*LOUISIANA*
*LBS. LOST 40*

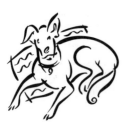

**THE BIGGEST ISSUE FOR ME** is eating out of boredom. When I am home alone for hours, I will always eat, just because I can. If I feel the urge, I always try to call a friend, take the dog for a walk, or just do something outside the apartment.

—*SARA WALKER*

• • • • • • • •

**MAKE SMALL, SLOW CHANGES,** like adding an evening walk to your day or having cut carrots in the fridge. If you deprive yourself too much, you won't make it.

—*NANCY MCBRIDE*
*NEW ORLEANS, LOUISIANA*
*LBS. LOST 40*

• • • • • • • •

**I REALLY ENJOY PRIA LOW CARB BARS.** By cutting them in half, they make a filling and tasty dessert. And, they are much better for you than a real dessert!

—*ANONYMOUS*
*NEW YORK, NEW YORK*
*LBS. LOST 20*

• • • • • • • •

**NEVER EAT CHIPS OR PRETZELS** from a bag. It's too easy to keep eating and eating, and pretty soon you've polished off a whole bag. Instead, measure out a portion into a bowl.

—*KAREN PHILLIPS*
*LANSING, ILLINOIS*
*LBS. LOST 42*

• • • • • • • •

**WHEN YOU ARE DONE EATING,** get up and do something active. Take the dog for a walk or just walk around the block. It aids digestion and makes you feel fuller later.

—*G.L.*
*NEW YORK, NEW YORK*
*LBS. LOST 15*

**SNACKING IS DEFINITELY ALLOWED.** The more often you eat throughout the day, the better your metabolism will be. Instead of metabolizing a meal, then shutting off, your metabolism will stay active throughout the day and help you burn more calories. Six small meals a day can often be better for dieters than three larger meals.

—BOB HOLDEN
NEW YORK, NEW YORK

· · · · · · · · ·

" Don't tell anyone about your diet. You are guaranteed to have someone try and talk you out of it. They'll wave ice-cream cake in front of your face and sing 'Na-na, na-na-na.' "

—L.S.
NEW YORK, NEW YORK
LBS. LOST 15

· · · · · · · · ·

**ABSOLUTELY NO BUTTER.** It's one of those little things that people don't think is going to hurt all that much, but it really adds up. It's something that many people are unwilling to cut out of their diet, but you would be surprised at the taste of some of the substitutes they have on the market today. You just can't have any real butter.

—JEFFREY SMITH
HARMONY, PENNSYLVANIA
LBS. LOST 15

Make sure that your house is de-junked (free of junk food) before you start a weight-loss program.

—KATIE
OREM, UTAH
LBS. LOST 45

# MORE ON METABOLISM: IT'S THE HORMONES, HONEY

Hormones can be a major influence on your metabolism. If you are a woman between the ages of 35 and 55, you can attest to how difficult weight loss has become. The average age of menopause is 51. The 10-15 years prior to menopause is called perimenopause. Because you need estrogen to stay female, and your reproductive organs are producing less and less estrogen as perimenopause progresses, the fat cells of the female body take on a larger role in the production of estrogen. Fat cells have always contributed to estrogen production, but during perimenopause the fat cells in the upper body, particularly the abdomen, start storing even more fat.  The average woman will find herself gaining at least 6 pounds during perimenopause, and if those pounds are all in the belly, even the slimmest will find her waistband growing tight.

**AT THE TIMES WHEN I REALLY** want to snack, I choose vegetables with a low-calorie, high-flavor dip like mustard or chipotle sauce. I find that satisfies me.

—*DAVID HUBBELL*
*KIRKLAND, WASHINGTON*
LBS. LOST *50*

. . . . . . . .

" Stay away from McDonald's. And Wendy's. And Burger King. Don't discriminate against any one fast-food restaurant chain: stay away from them all. "

—*EILEEN*
*PITTSBURGH, PENNSYLVANIA*
LBS. LOST *15*

. . . . . . . .

**DON'T SACRIFICE FLAVOR!** I love spicy foods, and one of my favorite snacks was chips and salsa. Now, I still enjoy the salsa, but on bell pepper strips instead. It's a double dose of vegetables.

—*DAPHNE*
*OREM, UTAH*
LBS. LOST *47*

. . . . . . . .

**IF I DRINK A LOT OF WATER** it makes me feel better about myself, and that makes it easier to stay away from the foods that I'm not supposed to have.

—*CORIN*
*PAYSON, UTAH*
LBS. LOST *41*

**IF YOU LIKE ICE CREAM,** as I do, you can't have it in the house. I don't care if your husband or your kids like ice cream and are not dieting: It's just too tempting. They will have to learn to live without it if they want to see a slimmer, trimmer you.

—COLLEEN JASTRZEBSKI
BULGER, PENNSYLVANIA
LBS. LOST *12*

• • • • • • • •

66 Don't go to the grocery store when you are hungry; you will buy what you are craving at the moment. 99

—G. COMPEAN
RIO MEDINA, TEXAS

• • • • • • • •

**DON'T DEVELOP AN AFFINITY** for breakfast tacos made with lard, don't move to the suburbs where you will never have the opportunity to walk again, and don't get an office job where you will spend 50 hours a week on your rear.

—ANONYMOUS
HELOTES, TEXAS
HAS GAINED A FEW POUNDS

• • • • • • • •

**TEMPTATION IS THE ROOT OF ALL DIETING EVIL:** Kill it at the source. Stay away from the supermarket aisles that carry junk food. You have no business venturing down them. And for God's sake, steer clear of the bakery!

—DON RODGERS
PITTSBURGH, PENNSYLVANIA
*9*

Take a bite and then put down your utensils until you swallow. That'll slow you down.

—ANONYMOUS
STRONGSVILLE, OHIO
LBS. LOST *21*

**WHEN NUTS ARE INCLUDED IN A RECIPE,** chop them finely and you will only need about half of what the recipe calls for. No one will ever know what's missing. After all, it is the taste you are after, not the extra calories.

—SUSIE GALVEZ
RICHMOND, VIRGINIA
LBS. LOST *121*

• • • • • • • •

**DON'T FORGET TO COUNT** the calories in soda. I used to drink at least three Mountain Dews a day. That's the equivalent of about three candy bars! I switched to Diet Mountain Dew. I admit that it doesn't taste as good, but it saves a lot of calories.

—SUE SIFFORD
SIKESTON, MISSOURI
LBS. LOST *15*

• • • • • • • •

**FIND REPLACEMENT SNACKS.** I have diabetes, so for me weight loss has to last forever. I may crave sweets, but sugar is out of the question because it gives me terrible headaches, so I snack on things like popcorn instead.

—WENDY
CEDAR HILLS, UTAH
LBS. LOST *45*

• • • • • • • •

**NUTS ARE GREAT TO SATISFY HUNGER.** If you're like me, though, portion them out. I once bought a whole bag and put it in my desk drawer. That did not work; they were gone really fast! Now I bring a serving size—10 to 15 nuts—to work each day in a plastic bag.

—CATHY
SPRINGVILLE, UTAH
LBS. LOST *48*

## A BIG GIGGLE

Ten to 15 minutes of hearty laughter burns fifty calories—about the same as a 13-minute walk at a quick pace.

# SMOKE AND MIRRORS

**TALK TO A FASHION PERSON** at any department store. They can help you find the clothes that are slimming for your body type. I've done this many times. I have several pairs of slacks that I wear that cause people to ask me, "Are you losing weight?"

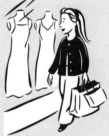

> —*DEB MORGAN*
> *FAIR OAKS RANCH, TEXAS*
> *LBS. LOST 60*

* * * * * * * * *

**WEARING THE RIGHT UNDERWEAR,** like support pantyhose or minimizing bras, helps a little. I also try to wear dark colors and nothing too tight, so little bulges here and there go unnoticed.

> —*V.B.*
> *NEW YORK, NEW YORK*
> *LBS. LOST 20*

* * * * * * * * *

**BIG BOOBS JUST MAKE WOMEN LOOK BIGGER** in general. But a good bra goes a really long way towards making you look better. The real danger—the thing that will make you look the fattest—is if your boobs are big and aren't up high enough. Hike up those bra straps! Buy a sports bra that's a size or two too small. You'll be amazed at the difference.

> —*B.R.*
> *CHAPEL HILL, NORTH CAROLINA*
> *LBS. LOST 30*

* * * * * * * * *

**IT'S FUNNY, BUT WHENEVER** I stand up straight people ask if I've lost weight!

> —*J.S.*
> *IOWA CITY, IOWA*
> *LBS. LOST 25*

**SEEK OUT HEALTHIER ALTERNATIVES** to foods that you crave. For example, the food I crave the most is ice cream. I find that I can substitute similar things that are lower in calories and carbs, such as ice milk, and still satisfy that craving.

—*CORIN*
*PAYSON, UTAH*
LBS. LOST *41*

. . . . . . . .

**IF I'M STUDYING,** I'll study till a certain time, then I'll have a healthy snack. It's a reward for getting the work done. That way I'm not sitting there eating all night.

—*VANESSA*
*MILWAUKEE, WISCONSIN*

. . . . . . . .

**I DRINK AN AWFUL LOT OF WATER**—about two liters a day. Yes, there are often times when I'm dashing to the bathroom, but the water helps keep my hunger at bay.

—*MARY*
*ALLENTOWN, PENNSYLVANIA*
LBS. LOST *25*

. . . . . . . .

**DON'T WORK NEAR A DONUT SHOP.** I worked near a Dunkin' Donuts, a Europa Café shop, and a bakery. Every day, I had to walk past the smell of donuts baking. I gained 10 pounds.

—*SARAH SPARKS*
*WASHINGTON, D.C.*
LBS. LOST *6*

. . . . . . . .

**IF YOU'VE GOT TO HAVE CARBS,** eat them early in the day. That way, you've got the whole day to burn them off.

—*ANONYMOUS*
*AIEA, HAWAII*
LBS. LOST *15*

Chew sugarless gum. I'm a nibbler when I cook: Now that I chew gum, it keeps me from nibbling.

—*KAREN PHILLIPS*
*LANSING, ILLINOIS*
LBS. LOST *42*

**Give up things you can do without. When I need to lose weight I stop my nightly Tastykake-after-dinner ritual.**

*—JOHN R. BRIGHT*
*ALLENTOWN,*
*PENNSYLVANIA*
*LBS. LOST 20*

**EAT A HEALTHIER VERSION OF FOODS** you can't give up, like pizza. I make English muffin pizzas with sauce, cheese, mushrooms, and pepperoni from the deli. It's about 300 calories less than the Papa John's version!

*—J.S.*
*IOWA CITY, IOWA*
*LBS. LOST 25*

• • • • • • • •

**I'VE MADE A VOW** not to be the family dog: I won't finish eating what my kids leave on their plates. A quarter of a grilled cheese sandwich goes into the trash.

*—CHARLOTTE PARKER*
*DES MOINES, IOWA*
*LBS. LOST 3*

# You Can do it: Sticking with it and Keeping it Off

*A*t some point on your weight-loss journey, you'll probably wonder what's taking so long, and question whether you'll ever reach your goal. Just keep this in mind: all those extra pounds did not appear overnight, so they're not going to disappear overnight. For tips on sticking with your weight-loss program, and strategies for keeping the weight off for life, read on.

**DON'T TAKE YOURSELF TOO SERIOUSLY.** If you fall off the diet wagon, laugh at yourself for being human and try again.

—*ANONYMOUS*
*DOUGLASVILLE, GEORGIA*
*LBS. LOST 10*

**FOR ME, IT'S EASIER TO *KEEP* IT OFF THAN *TAKE* IT OFF.**

—*ANONYMOUS*
*PITTSBURGH, PENNSYLVANIA*

**Stick with it. I believe that most diets die an early death because dieters expect to see results right away. It just doesn't work that way. These things take time.**

—*Cindy Rodgers*
*Pittsburgh,*
*Pennsylvania*
*lbs. lost 12*

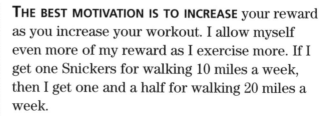

**THE BEST MOTIVATION IS TO INCREASE** your reward as you increase your workout. I allow myself even more of my reward as I exercise more. If I get one Snickers for walking 10 miles a week, then I get one and a half for walking 20 miles a week.

—*Andrea Weigand*
*Woodworth, Ohio*
*lbs. lost 11*

. . . . . . . .

**GIVE YOURSELF CREDIT** for the good things you are doing (exercising every day), don't focus only on the bad things you're doing (eating Chinese food). The key is positive thinking and taking small steps to creating good habits.

—*Kate O.*
*Philadelphia, Pennsylvania*
*lbs. lost 10*

. . . . . . . .

**FOCUS ON WHAT YOU HAVE ACCOMPLISHED,** not what lies ahead. If you have 150 pounds to lose and have lost 25, focus on the weight lost, not the 125 pounds you still have left. When I was losing weight, I could not think in terms of the total amount of weight I had to lose; it was unbearable. Focusing on the positive made it seem possible. I used this method all the way down the scale.

—*Patricia Michener*
*West Grove, Pennsylvania*
*lbs. lost 146*

. . . . . . . .

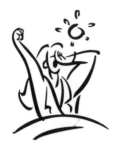

**WORK ON YOUR DIET DAY BY DAY.** Instead of saying, "Gee, I have to lose so many pounds," I say, "This is the day I'm going to eat sensibly and see what happens." The next day, I get up and say, "OK, I'm going to continue to eat sensibly."

—*Susan*
*Atlanta, Georgia*
*lbs. lost 40*

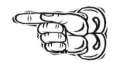

**ONCE YOU ACHIEVE YOUR GOAL,** you cannot revert to your old way of life: Those days are over. Too many people lose the weight and then start right back in with the sweets. You have to understand that you are a new person. Those old lifestyle choices are behind you, never to be seen again.

—*ANONYMOUS*
*EAST PALESTINE, OHIO*
*LBS. LOST 13*

- - - - - - - - -

" Do things to keep your hands busy—that way you can't eat. When I was learning to knit, I realized that it kept me from snacking. I didn't get as hungry because my mind was occupied, and it was too hard to set my knitting down to get a snack. "

—*AMY*
*ALBURTIS, PENNSYLVANIA*

- - - - - - - - -

**USE TOOLS THAT WILL HELP YOU LOSE.** I got a digital scale that weighs in .2-pound increments, and I use it every day. That's what broke my potato-chip habit. I'd eat a little bag and be up a pound and a half the next day.

—*ANONYMOUS*
*NEW YORK, NEW YORK*
*LBS. LOST 17*

# THE PART-TIME DIET

Surviving a diet is doable; however, living on a diet is damn near impossible. I tried to live on them all: Atkins, South Beach, fasting, cabbage soup. I was usually successful for about two weeks at a time, but by the third week the diet was over and my plan to swear off carbs and sugar was shot.

My suggestion: Everything in moderation—including diets! That suggestion is usually applied to situations in which we are faced with dessert menus, wine lists, and delicious, fresh bread baskets. But what about minimizing your dieting time as well? The need for dieting will diminish if you choose to stay on top of what you eat on a daily basis and commit to healthy eating 80 percent of the time. M&M's and wine must be allowed  on certain days.

—M.J.F.
NEW YORK, NEW YORK
LBS. LOST 5-10

THE ONLY THING THAT HAS EVER kept me at it when I most felt like quitting was the realization that I was adding days on to the end of my life. If you think about it like that it's easy to keep going. Just think: there is a day in the future when you will die. But if you eat right, exercise, and take better care of yourself you can definitely push that date back. That's a fact. If that's not enough motivation for you then you're hopeless.

—G.M.
CUMBERLAND, MARYLAND
LBS. LOST 17

**FIND NEW THINGS TO MOTIVATE YOU.** I used to go into this restaurant where a cute, young, foreign busboy worked. We were casual friends. He stopped working there for about a year, and when he came back I walked in the door and he cried, "You look so wonderful! Really great!" His comment made me realize I didn't want to gain the weight back. People really do notice and care. Remembering this moment is powerful motivation whenever I'm tempted to stop my diet.

> —E.C.
> NEW YORK, NEW YORK
> LBS. LOST 20

**NEVER ENOUGH?**

Forty-six percent of Americans who are on a diet, and have already lost some weight, say they want to lose 21 to 30 pounds more.

• • • • • • • •

**THE TRICK IS TO INCORPORATE** your healthy eating and exercise in a daily routine. If you take a diet seriously and exercise regularly, you will see the results you need to keep you motivated. If you slack off and tell yourself it isn't working, then you are talking yourself out of it. Find a plan that you can stick to for the long haul.

> —ANONYMOUS
> SONOMA, CALIFORNIA

• • • • • • • •

**THERE'S ALWAYS THE INITIAL EUPHORIA** when you start a new diet—you feel powerful and in control. But then there's that guilt when you (inevitably, of course) fall off the track. That's the point when you usually sabotage everything and go down in a blaze of Häagen-Dazs! You need to think ahead and plan how you'll pick yourself up after you fall. I wrote myself a letter, which I re-read when I need to.

> —SHELLEY GLADSTONE
> ATLANTA, GEORGIA
> LBS. LOST 15

Every time I get an urge to eat lettuce or celery or something like that, I grab an Oreo cookie and lie down until the urge passes!

—*ANONYMOUS*
*DOUGLASVILLE,*
*GEORGIA*
*LBS. LOST 10*

**CONCENTRATE ON FEELING GOOD** and being healthy instead of what the scale says. Even though I had a successful career and loving family, I felt like a failure. I let my extra weight erode my self-image. I had tried every diet. Finally, I realized that I was not the problem—the diets were.

—*MAYTAL YARON*
*LOS ANGELES, CALIFORNIA*
*LBS. LOST 15*

• • • • • • • •

**CONSISTENCY AND ROUTINE** are crucial. When I'm working out and getting into a routine, I'm completely into it. But if I take a few days off, order pizza, and sit on the couch, I fall off the wagon.

—*J. LEWIS*
*PHILADELPHIA, PENNSYLVANIA*

• • • • • • • •

**DON'T BE HARD ON YOURSELF** while you are losing weight. Allow yourself to slip occasionally, but have the courage to go back to your eating plan. It can really be frustrating when you hit a plateau, but that's all the more reason to allow yourself the small setbacks. The more I worried about the scale and the weight loss, the less I lost. Relax and the results will come!

—*KAREN BUFFUM*
*ROUND ROCK, TEXAS*
*LBS. LOST 25*

• • • • • • • •

**DON'T LET UP WHEN YOU START** to have a little success and you lose a couple of pounds. You have to keep your foot on the pedal. Some people see the first fruits of their labor and think they can lapse. I would lose 10 pounds, and then I would say, "Well, I can have a piece of cake." But it comes back just as quickly as it left.

—*TERRI MASTELL*
*PETERSBURG, OHIO*
*LBS. LOST 10*

# BY THE BOOK

One of the most helpful things I've ever done while dieting was this: After I'd lost 20 pounds, I piled 20 pounds of encyclopedias on the scale, then picked them all up and walked around the house with them for about 10 minutes. I was exhausted! It vividly demonstrated to me what it felt like for my body to be carting around all that extra weight. Even an extra 10 pounds will cause fatigue.

Regardless of how much weight you've lost, this is a valuable way to reinforce the good you're doing and to help keep you on track.

—CAROL
LOS ANGELES, CALIFORNIA
LBS. LOST 25

**DON'T EXPECT TOO MUCH** of yourself right off the bat. It took you a while to develop all your bad eating habits and it will take you a little while to create new, healthy habits. If you feel weak and allow yourself a candy bar, that doesn't mean that you have failed. Try again.

—DIANE ROSE SMITH
HARMONY, PENNSYLVANIA
LBS. LOST 10

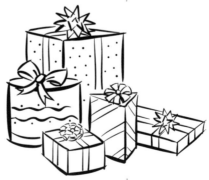

**YOU NEED PATIENCE MORE THAN WILLPOWER** to be successful. To lose a pound of fat, you need a calorie deficit of 3,500 calories. That's not going to happen overnight. Remember, if it's fast, it won't last.

—*EVELYN RICHARDS*
*SUMMERVILLE, SOUTH CAROLINA*
*LBS. LOST 65*

* * * * * * * *

" Use food as motivation. The first meal I eat after I've reached my target weight will be the best meal I've ever eaten. "

—*MARY ZAYCHICK*
*CUMBERLAND, MARYLAND*
*LBS. LOST 10*

* * * * * * * *

**DON'T FOCUS SO MUCH ON DIETING,** but on discipline. When you learn how to control your physical appetite, you have the ability to change your world; you will have become the master of your feelings, and will have learned to see beyond the tangible. Just keep telling yourself every time you refuse a piece of pie or chocolate cake that you are one step closer to becoming your own personal revolutionary!

—*SHELLIE R. WARREN*
*NASHVILLE, TENNESSEE*
*LBS. LOST 15*

**YOU KNOW THE FEELING:** You worked hard for weeks and then in one moment, you've eaten it all back, and more. Don't beat yourself up about it. It's important to put the brakes on the binge as soon as you can. Plan ahead of time how you're going to handle a slip. Successful dieters aren't perfect all the time. (And if they say they are, they're lying or really neurotic, and we don't want them as our friends anyway.) I handle a slip by writing in a food diary religiously for the following week. That gets me back on track fast.

—*LORI B.*
*CHARLESTON, SOUTH CAROLINA*
*LBS. LOST 10*

**DON'T GET DISCOURAGED.** It just takes time. I did it in five-pound increments because the 20 pounds I wanted to lose was such a large, unattainable goal. Setting little achievements along the way made the goal seem more attainable. When I lost two pounds, I would get excited because I was almost at five pounds.

—*R.M.*
*CAMBRIDGE, MASSACHUSETTS*
*LBS. LOST 14*

# HOLDING FIRM

Some time ago, 95 percent of dieters who succeeded in losing weight gained it all back—but that's no longer true! Thanks to advances in the treatment of obesity over the years, more and more people are losing weight and keeping it off.

# TEMPTATION TIME?

**SEVEN P.M.:** That's because I teach a yoga class at five o'clock, and I'll be hungry for supper before the class even starts. I make sure to snack on vegetables, maybe with some fat-free dip, before I leave for class. I keep vegetables cut up and batched in Ziploc bags in my refrigerator.

—*JOAN RAINWATER*
*WATERVILLE, OHIO*
*LBS. LOST 37*

**TEN A.M.:** I usually get up for work at six thirty and eat a small break-fast. That will hold me over until about nine thirty or ten o'clock, when my stomach usually starts making enough noise to disturb my coworkers in the cubicles next to me. The bad part is that we have to take lunch at twelve thirty, so I know I still have two and a half hours to go before I can have any food. I've started keeping some rice cakes in my desk. They are nasty, but it's better than nothing.

—*TRACY MOLLICA*
*YOUNGSTOWN, OHIO*
*LBS. LOST 9*

**MIDNIGHT:** Oh man, I get off work late (midnight some nights) and I am hungry! And I want my cookies, and pizza, or cheesy tortillas, so bad.

—*J.S.*
*IOWA CITY, IOWA*
*LBS. LOST 25*

**AFTER DINNER:** I have to remember not to just sit at the computer and continually munch. I try to save some fruit and popcorn for the evening, and I drink a lot of herbal tea then, too.

—*DEB WUNDER*
*BROOKLYN, NEW YORK*
*LBS. LOST 36*

**TWO THIRTY IN THE AFTERNOON:** It's that time where that little salad you had for lunch is gone and dinner is still hours away. The candy machine at the office seems to be calling your name. I'd bring in a piece of fruit or some rice cakes, but I can't say that I didn't still hear the Reese's Peanut Butter Cups calling me.

—*WILLIAM GREEN*
*FROSTBURG, MARYLAND*
*LBS. LOST 9*

. . . . . . . . .

**NOON:** Lunch is the meal that gives me fits. I actually had to quit the diet because Mickey D's was so close to my office, and I only get a half hour for lunch.

—*SANDRA MONROE*
*CUMBERLAND, MARYLAND*
*LBS. LOST 50*

. . . . . . . . .

**EIGHT TO NINE P.M.:** I talk on the phone or take a bubble bath to distract myself from food. If it gets unbearable, I just call it a night and go to sleep early. I also have the occasional three to four p.m. craving, and I just have some coffee.

—*V.B.*
*NEW YORK, NEW YORK*
*LBS. LOST 20*

. . . . . . . . .

**MORNING:** I'd eat late at night and then be really hungry in the morning. But when I stopped eating late at night, it gave me a sense of control, and I discovered that I'm no longer so hungry in the mornings.

—*LEAH F.*
*SUFFERN, NEW JERSEY*

**GOOD WORK!**

Twenty-four percent of Americans on a diet report that they have lost up to five pounds, 22 percent say they have lost between five and 10 pounds, and 19 percent say they have lost between 11 and 20 pounds.

**IT'S IMPORTANT TO MIX THINGS UP** so that you don't get bored. I set a goal for myself that I would change my eating and exercise habits, and it worked great—for six months. Then I hit a plateau and was stuck at the same weight for two months. At the time, the YMCA was offering classes in spinning. So I tried it. It was fun, but even better, the change broke me through my weight-loss plateau. Within two weeks I'd lost another three pounds. Now, there's another new class: boot camp. I think I'll give it a shot!

—*JOAN RAINWATER*
*WATERVILLE, OHIO*
*LBS. LOST 37*

. . . . . . . . .

**THE KEY TO MAINTAINING YOUR NEW,** lower weight once you reach your goal is to understand that the whole process is a lifelong change. The old you, with the bad eating habits, is gone forever. If you go into a diet focused solely on losing 20 pounds and giving no thought to what comes after, then you are doomed to regain the weight.

—*WALTER HUGHES*
*CLEVELAND, OHIO*
*LBS. LOST 22*

. . . . . . . . .

**EVERY TIME I TRY TO STICK TO A DIET,** I end up cheating, no matter which plan it is. It took me a while to learn that I can't successfully lose weight when someone else dictates what I can eat and how much I should exercise. Instead, I put less pressure on myself and concentrate on making subtle changes. I eat less, but I won't count calories. I don't formally go to the gym, but I definitely take the stairs more. You'd be amazed at how these subtle changes can really add up.

—*L.E.*
*POMONA, CALIFORNIA*
*LBS. LOST 75*

**IF YOU LOSE SEVERAL POUNDS,** and several sizes, treat yourself to a shopping spree. Buying well-fitting clothes will not only make you feel great, but you will look better and be motivated to not gain the weight back. However, don't make the mistake of buying clothes that are too small, with the intention of fitting into them someday. This will just frustrate you.

—*DEBBIE*
*TULSA, OKLAHAMA*
*LBS. LOST 50*

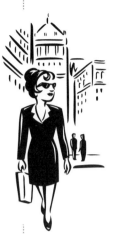

• • • • • • • • •

**WHEN I'D REACH MY GOAL WEIGHT** on a diet, I'd eat everything as my reward. I kept gaining weight, and honestly didn't know why. I joined a 12-step program and heard what now seems obvious: Your metabolism slows down when you put smaller amounts of food into your body, so that when you eat a lot again, you'll gain more weight than you started off with.

—*DEEDEE MELMET*
*SONOMA, CALIFORNIA*
*LBS. LOST 50*

• • • • • • • • •

**I USED TO TORMENT MYSELF** (and I mean serious psychological abuse here) by making myself try on my "skinny" jeans at least once a week. I wouldn't let myself buy new clothes until I lost weight. And every time I'd pass a mirror, I'd give myself a venomous talk about how disgusting I looked. And the sick thing is—I'm actually a pretty nice person! I finally realized that the constant put-downs were only making me crave more chocolate and undermining my self-esteem. I talk to myself now like I talk to my good girlfriends and try to be supportive, encouraging and positive. (And I threw out those jeans!)

—*EVELYN RICHARDS*
*SUMMERVILLE, SOUTH CAROLINA*
*LBS. LOST 65*

Don't let your diet rule your life. It's not worth it to diet so compulsively that you can't enjoy yourself.

—*MARY BRIGHT*
*ALLENTOWN,*
*PENNSYLVANIA*

# SUCCESS STORIES

*Here's an inspirational collection: Happy moments and success stories of people who have won their battles of the bulge. May you count yourself among the weight-loss winners very soon!*

**ONE OF THE HAPPIEST MOMENTS** for me was hearing my daughter tell her friends, "My mom looks like a model."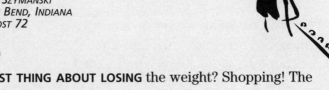

> —*DIANE SZYMANSKI*
> *SOUTH BEND, INDIANA*
> *LBS. LOST 72*

**THE VERY BEST THING ABOUT LOSING** the weight? Shopping! The first thing I bought was a pair of low-rise jeans.

> —*JOAN RAINWATER*
> *WATERVILLE, OHIO*
> *LBS. LOST 37*

**I REMEMBER THIS PAIR OF PANTS** I bought in my last fat summer. They had been the most flattering things I owned. One spring day, I got out those pants to wear: they were almost three sizes too big for me. They wouldn't even stay up. It was the most amazing feeling, looking down at that empty space in the pants that used to be extra me.

> —*B.R.*
> *CHAPEL HILL, NORTH CAROLINA*
> *LBS. LOST 30*

**LOSING WEIGHT IS INDESCRIBABLE;** everything changes. Buying clothes from "normal stores" was the first milestone. It's an incredible feeling. Then there are things that people never think about that make you happy, like your hips not touching each side of the chair, putting on a L or XL T-shirt.

> —*ROBERT DUBLAN JR.*
> *NEW ORLEANS, LOUISIANA*
> *LBS. LOST 120*

**I LOST QUITE A BIT OF WEIGHT** and the culmination was my 50th birthday. My husband threw a huge party for me at a swanky steakhouse, which was Atkins-correct. Before the party I went shopping with my daughter, who is a wicked fashionista, and we found a bright red dress that was perfect for me. I wore it to the party and looked really good!

—MARIAH
TORONTO, ONTARIO, CANADA
LOST 3 SIZES

• • • • • • • • •

**WHEN I WAS ON MY WAY DOWN,** I could just taste what it was going to be like when I was at my ideal weight. I knew I was going to make it, and I was so excited! I had these great episodes in changing rooms where clothes actually slid onto my body (instead of me having to tug them up).

—CECE BLASE
ALAMEDA, CALIFORNIA
LBS. LOST 25

• • • • • • • • •

**I BUMPED INTO AN ACQUAINTANCE** I hadn't seen for almost a year, and he excitedly remarked, "My God, what did you do? You look great!"

—SYLVIA W. STODDARD
HOLLY HILL, FLORIDA
LBS. LOST 65

• • • • • • • • •

**I PICKED MY MOM UP AT THE AIRPORT.** We hadn't seen each other for a few months, and when my mom saw me, her face dropped in surprise. The expression on her face made all of my weight-loss struggles worth it! My mom hadn't seen me this slim since my freshman year, and she, more than anyone, knew how much I had struggled with my weight over the years.

—ZORA ANDRICH
LAMBERTVILLE, NEW JERSEY
LBS. LOST 20

**IF YOU GO OFF YOUR DIET** for a day or two, don't think, "Well, I might as well give up." You can—and will—bounce back. But if you use a little weakness as an excuse to totally go off your program, you're in for trouble. Everyone fails from time to time.

> —*ANNE SMALLEY*
> *WOODBURY, NEW JERSEY*
> *LBS. LOST* 10

• • • • • • • •

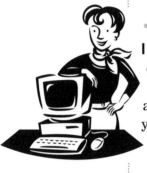

**I HAVE A "DIETER'S GROUP"** of four women. We log our calories every day and send them to each other via e-mail. This way, we're more accountable. Instead of putting those Oreo cookies in your mouth before bedtime, you think, "I'll have to report it."

> —*CECILIA CARSON*
> *COLUMBIA, MISSOURI*
> *LBS. LOST* 11

• • • • • • • •

**TO MOTIVATE MYSELF TO WORK OUT** and eat healthier I tell myself the following: "You like to have sex. The better shape you are in, the better off you are in that department." Therefore, sex is my driving point!

> —*J.S.*
> *IOWA CITY, IOWA*
> *LBS. LOST* 25

• • • • • • • •

**NO FLUCTUATION IS OK.** If you start saying stuff like, "Oh, it's only one pound," then suddenly that one pound becomes two, then three, then four. I immediately nip any weight gain in the bud. I'm a lifetime member of Weight Watchers, and in the maintenance stage they only allow a two-pound fluctuation before they start charging you money. What a great incentive to stay on track.

> —*S. BILBY*
> *ARVADA, COLORADO*
> *LBS. LOST* 20

**I THINK I'LL BE WRITING DOWN** what I eat for a very long time. Even on the days where I'm keeping mental track, I end up jotting it down later. You can't fall into the old, "Well, I screwed up the whole day already so why not finish it off with a bang." Each meal is a choice, and chance to start over.

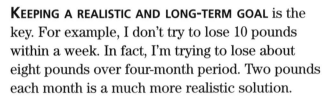

> —ANONYMOUS
> LOS ANGELES, CALIFORNIA
> LBS. LOST 20

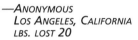

**KEEPING A REALISTIC AND LONG-TERM GOAL** is the key. For example, I don't try to lose 10 pounds within a week. In fact, I'm trying to lose about eight pounds over four-month period. Two pounds each month is a much more realistic solution.

> —ANONYMOUS
> HARTFORD, CONNECTICUT
> LBS. LOST 4

**THE EASIEST WAY TO SURVIVE** a diet is to forgive yourself when you veer from it. If you find yourself eating junk, then at least let yourself enjoy it. The eating of the junk is not the problem. Beating yourself up for it is the problem.

> —MICHAEL ALPERSTEIN
> PETALUMA, CALIFORNIA
> LBS. LOST 5

**LET YOURSELF GO ONCE A WEEK.** Never has food tasted so good and put a smile on my face as when I was following Weight Watchers and eating next to nothing for two weeks. My girlfriend and I went out and had a big meal—a hundred times more than I'd eaten in the past two weeks—and each bite tasted as if I was in heaven.

> —BUZZ ORR
> EVANSTON, ILLINOIS
> LBS. LOST 15

**ALLOW YOURSELF SOME LITTLE TREAT** to look forward to each day. That's my happiest moment, that time in the evening when I have my little treat. Even if it's just something like one cookie or a little glass of chocolate milk, it makes all the difference in the world. Don't go crazy and let yourself eat a bag of microwave popcorn, but one little cookie is not that bad if it keeps you on track.

—*DEB PRZYWARTY*
*IRWIN, PENNSYLVANIA*
*LBS. LOST 28*

. . . . . . . . .

**HAVE YOUR CLOTHES TAILORED.** You'll be excited to see your old clothes look new and better, and you won't want to gain the weight back after spending all the money on alterations. I had a ton of my clothes altered a year ago. The tailor was pinning the inseam, and she said, "How did you lose it in the butt?" It was so funny; and so nice to be asked for advice!

—*WENDY*
*SAN FRANCISCO, CALIFORNIA*
*LBS. LOST 17*

. . . . . . . . .

**IT'S DIFFICULT TO STAY MOTIVATED** once you reach your goal and start reaping all the compliments. It's so easy to say to yourself, "I look great; let's eat!" But you just need to remind yourself what you looked like before, and the effort it took to get where you are now. A "before" and "after" picture on the fridge might be a good reminder!

—*MIRI GREIDI*
*RA'ANANA, ISRAEL*
*LBS. LOST 53*

# More Wisdom: Good Stuff That Doesn't Fit Anywhere Else

T*he journey to a new, slimmer you is filled with ups and downs. As a reward for all your hard work and self-deprivation, we offer you an extra helping of advice to motivate you along the way.*

**LEARN TO LOVE YOURSELF** before you lose the weight. Otherwise, you go from being fat and unhappy to being thin and unhappy.

> —CAROL SIMPSON
> WOODBURY, NEW JERSEY
> LBS. LOST 15

**REMEMBER, WE'RE SOPHISTICATED, DIVINELY DESIGNED ANIMALS. WE NEED VERY LITTLE FOOD TO SURVIVE.**

> —TOM W.
> LENOX,
> MASSACHUSETTS

**SOMETIMES IT'S HARD FOR PEOPLE** who have been heavy to accept compliments about their weight. If someone tells you how good you look, I think the best thing to say is a simple, "Thank you very much."

—MARY BRIGHT
ALLENTOWN, PENNSYLVANIA

• • • • • • • •

" Don't work in an office. All they do is order pizza, get birthday cake, and share chocolates and macadamia nuts from business trips. Plus, you sit at a desk all day. "

—L.S.
NEW YORK, NEW YORK
LBS. LOST 15

Any diet will work if you stick to it. Your attitude counts as much as the calories.

—JOSH KAYE
WINNIPEG,
MANITOBA,
CANADA
LBS. LOST 30

• • • • • • • •

**REALIZE THAT SOCIETY WANTS US** to be thin to support the multi-billion-dollar beauty, diet, and health industry. Without making you feel horrible about the way you look, how could gyms, salons, plastic surgeons, and countless other businesses make money? In order to preserve your happiness, you must know that you are doing this for the right reasons—for your body, your health, and your well-being.

—ANDREA MANITSAS

**I HAVE LOST 110 POUNDS.** It has taken me about six years, but it was well worth the wait. The main advice is to be strong. You must want to achieve a goal no matter what it takes. You have to want it with all of your being, and *you* have to come first. I lost the first 60 on my own by exercising, and then I joined Weight Watchers and lost the rest in about three years. I am a completely different person now, inside and out. I eat mostly healthy foods and work out three days a week, mostly jogging. You can do anything you want to do if you really *want* to.

—*RACHEL COSSMAN*
*SOUTH BEND, INDIANA*
*LBS. LOST 110*

If you want to be thin, don't let your wife have kids. My brother put on sympathy weight for each of his wife's four pregnancies, and he still hasn't got it off. She looks great, though.

—*BOB SCHULTZ*
*HOPEWELL*
*TOWNSHIP,*
*PENNSYLVANIA*
*LBS. LOST 20*

**A TRUE DIET BECOMES** a spiritual transformation. It's not simply your grocery list that must change, but your relationship to food in general; what it means to you; the role that it occupies in your life. Overall, we have given food too much importance in our lives. It has become a comfort, companion, lover, enemy, and friend when, in fact, all it was intended to do is give us sustenance. I once read that when you can leave a thing, then you have mastered it: If you cannot leave it, then it has mastered you. Food has truly mastered this society, and we have become its slaves. This is no mistake.

—*OMO MISHA*
*NEW YORK, NEW YORK*

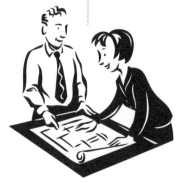

**GET A JOB** where you are on your feet all day. I care for the elderly, and I am very active. I walk all day. If I fancy something, I eat it—sweets, meat, anything.

—*DAWN O'DONNELL*
*YORKSHIRE, ENGLAND*

# TRUE OR FALSE?

*No answer key is provided: You already know the correct answers!*

1. If you order Diet Coke, it cancels out all the calories of that super-value meal.
2. Calories you drink don't count.
3. Ditto for calories you consume while standing up.
4. If you eat more than half of the pint of ice cream, you must finish it and hide the evidence.
5. Half the calories means you can eat twice as much.
6. Dr. Atkins? Was that the cute doctor on ER?

—*JENNIFER SHULL*
*NEW YORK, NEW YORK*

**MY FATHER USED TO USE A LINE** that I hardly ever paid attention to, until I was in my forties: Everything in moderation. That's the key. I've tried all sorts of diets, and it took me a long time to understand that if you exercise regularly and don't overindulge in anything, you can eat whatever you like.

—*DEBBIE REDDEN-BRUNELLO*
*TEMECULA, CALIFORNIA*
LBS. LOST *30*

If you want a sure-fire way to lose weight, try getting divorced. The stress of it will work wonders.

—*DAWN K.*
*READING,*
*PENNSYLVANIA*
LBS. LOST *25*

**DIETS DON'T WORK** because you talk yourself out of doing them. You say they're too expensive, or you think you can't *possibly* give up bread. The only time I dieted successfully was when I was in college and the food in the cafeteria was so bad I ate salads for six months. When you go through the cafeteria buffet and the roast beef has an iridescent blue sheen, you think, "Uh, no, let's go to the salad bar." Then, too, when I was 18 I had a zealot inside that said, "You have to look good." But now that I'm 55, I think, "This is the way it's going to be." I don't worry about my weight any more.

—*PEG*
*DENVER, COLORADO*

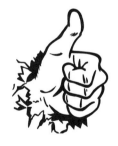

**THERE'S NO SUCH THING** as the perfect diet or the perfect exercise routine. Everything works well— for a while. But I've come to appreciate that while no one thing will completely solve my weight issues, it's still great to find something that solves 20% of the problem. Maybe something else will solve another 5% and something else even more. Eventually, you'll make it to 100%.

—*SHELLEY GLADSTONE*
*ATLANTA, GEORGIA*
LBS. LOST *15*

**I BELIEVE THAT DIETING** in and of itself is self-defeating; the real problem for people who need to lose weight is that the weight is symptomatic of something else, such as a psychological imbalance, or depression, or something missing in your life. Food is instant gratification. It's an addictive, easy-access, best-friend source of comfort. Dieting isn't healthy. People don't keep the weight off and there's a reason for that: We don't look for the reason we put the weight on in the first place. Instead of thinking about dieting, I think about getting healthy overall, whether I lose weight or not.

—V.M.
DENVER, COLORADO

. . . . . . . .

" Do not give up. Recognize that the sacrifice of pleasure in the short term will be returned tenfold in the end. "

—C.B.
FRANKLIN, MASSACHUSETTS
LBS. LOST 10-15

. . . . . . . .

**RELAX!** You only live your life once. Of course you should take care of yourself, but you should also enjoy the ride. Don't miss out on all of the fun.

—JENNIFER SHULL
NEW YORK, NEW YORK

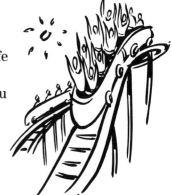

# NUGGETS

*Wisdom gathered from 55 years of dieting:*

1. Do not ignore any food group or food—just eat everything in moderation.
2. Do not throw your scales away, but do make them really hard to get to.
3. Become more active.
4. The sin is not going off the diet, it's not getting back on the diet quickly.

—*Roger Ghormley*
*Tulsa, Oklahoma*
*lbs. lost 75*

**DIETING IS ABOUT REASONING** with yourself and balancing your intake. Think about how often people overstuff themselves—a big meal at a restaurant, on holidays, at parties, or even at sporting events. There's always an excuse to overeat. Typically, when you overeat you're miserable; but somehow we find a way to reason with it. And you're equally miserable when you're hungry, but somehow it's impossible to justify letting yourself starve. I think you have to balance it out. If you're going to pig out one day, it might not be such a bad idea to eat a salad (no heavy dressing or cheese) for dinner the following day or two (or even all week).

—*N.L.*
*New York, New York*
*lbs. lost 10*

**Plan for the holidays by dieting two months ahead: you have to start losing weight before they get here.**

—*Rob Jones*
*Pittsburgh, Pennsylvania*
*lbs. lost 10*

**DON'T STRESS YOURSELF** out over a few pounds. You may think you need to lose weight, but you probably look a lot better to everyone else than you do to yourself.

—*Lori*
*Oklahoma City, Oklahoma*
*lbs. lost 20*

. . . . . . . . .

**THE PERFECT BODY IS UNATTAINABLE.** The closer you get to your initial goal, the more that goal morphs into something you can't have. Life is too short for deprivation; everything in balance, everything in moderation. Learning to feel good in your skin and listening to your body's hunger cues is far more important than following a strict diet or going along with a fad.

—*D.C.*

. . . . . . . . .

**The word "diet" in Greek means "a way of life," and my current diet really is a lifelong plan.**

—*Miri Greidi*
*Ra'anana, Israel*
*lbs. lost 53*

**I HATE THE TERM "DIETING"** because to me, it sounds like it's a temporary thing that you can stop doing once you've lost the weight. If you want to lose weight, you need to change your eating habits. That's tough, because these are habits you've probably had all of your life (and *everyone* has eating habits, no matter if they are underweight or overweight or at weight). Weight loss can be achieved once you think about what you're eating and how often you're eating and why you're eating. Many of us (myself included, prior to my weight loss) are not conscious of our daily food choices. But it is something to be aware of, especially in this day and age, when all of our portions have doubled within the last 30 years.

—*Margaret Steck*
*Seattle, Washington*
*lbs. lost 38*

# SPECIAL THANKS

Thanks to our intrepid "headhunters" for going out to find so many dieters from around the country with interesting advice to share:

Jamie Allen, Chief Headhunter

| | | |
|---|---|---|
| Jennifer Batog | Matt Villano | Ralph Fox |
| John Christensen | Sara Faiwell | Natasha Lambropoulos |
| Lisa Jaffe Hubbell | Shannon Hurd | Nicole Lessin |
| Ken McCarthy | Joanne Wolfe | Andrea Syrtash |
| Heather Leonard | Pippin Ross | Sara Walker |
| Besha Rodell | Jade Walker | |
| Connie Farrow | Jennifer Byrne | |

Thanks, too, to our editorial advisor Anne Kostick. And thanks to our assistant, Miri Greidi, for her yeoman's work at keeping us all organized, and for losing 53 pounds in the process.

The real credit for this book, of course, goes to all the people whose experiences and collective wisdom make up this guide. There are too many of you to thank individually, of course, but you know who you are.

# CREDITS

Page 2: "What is Obesity?" American Obesity Association, AOA Fact Sheets.

Page 7: The Center for the Study of Anorexia and Bulimia.

Page 8: "What is Obesity?" American Obesity Association, AOA Fact Sheets.

Page 10: "Numbers," *Time*, March 7, 2005.

Page 16: *www.guinnessworldrecords.com.*

Page 18: "Exercise and weight loss," MedlinePlus, Medical Encyclopedia.

Pages 24-25: "Lose by Gaining a New Lifestyle," by Joan Morris, The Diet Club, *Contra Costa Times*, June 21, 2005.

Page 26: "10 Things to Do when Your Diet's Not That Into You" by Stephanie Allmon, Fort Worth *Star-Telegram*, June 20, 2005.

Page 28: "Statistics Related to Overweight and Obesity," National Institute of Diabetes and Digestive and Kidney Diseases, Weight-control Information Network.

Page 31: "Obesity in the U.S.," American Obesity Association, AOA Fact Sheets.

Page 34: "Why Are You Overweight? The Inside Scoop On Dieting," Fat Loss 4 Idiots, *www.fatloss4idiots.com.*

Page 38: "The NPD's New Dieting Monitor Tracks America's Dieting Habits," NPD Foodworld, May 3, 2004.

Page 43: "The NPD's New Dieting Monitor Tracks America's Dieting Habits," NPD Foodworld, May 3, 2004.

Page 47: "Americans May Be Finding Balance in Their Eating Patterns," NPD Foodworld, October 13, 2004.

Page 56: "The NPD's New Dieting Monitor Tracks America's Dieting Habits," NPD Foodworld, April 5, 2004.

Page 57: "Are the Clues to Diet Success in Your Genes?" by Hilary MacGregor, *LA Times*, April 11, 2005.

Page 60: "The NPD's New Dieting Monitor Tracks America's Dieting Habits," NPD Foodworld, May 3, 2004.

Page 69: "Intelligence Report," by Lyric Wallwork Winik, *Parade* Magazine, March 7, 2004.

Page 70: "Crazy for Chocolate, Why Do I Crave Chocolate?" by Elizabeth Somer, MA, RD, WebMD, July 16, 2001.

Page 75: "Homemade Dessert Disappearing From the Dinner Table," NPD Foodworld, September 16, 2003.

Page 78: "U.S. Food Supply Providing More Food and Calories," by Judy Putman, *Food Review*, Volume 22, Issue 3.

Page 83: "Men's Top Health Threats: Mostly Preventable" by MayoClinic.com, MSN Health & Fitness.

Page 84: "Why it's hard to eat well and be active in America today," Center for Science in the Public Interest.

Page 87: "5 A Day: Fruit and Vegetable of the Month," Department of Health and Human Services, Centers for Disease Control and Prevention.

Page 89: "5 A Day: Fruit and Vegetable of the Month," Department of Health and Human Services, Centers for Disease Control and Prevention.

Page 96: Department of Health and Human Services, Centers for Disease Control and Prevention.

Page 97: "Overweight and Obesity: Frequently Asked Questions," Department of Health and Human Services, Centers for Disease Control and Prevention.

Page 97: Journal of Nutrition, volume 134, pages 3021-3025

Page 99: "Overweight and Obesity: Frequently Asked Questions," Department of Health and Human Services, Centers for Disease Control and Prevention.

Page 100: "Sales of diet soda could eclipse regular in a decade," J.M. Hirsch, *Associated Press*, December 21, 2004.

Page 101: "Overweight and Obesity: Frequently Asked Questions," Department of Health and Human Services, Centers for Disease Control and Prevention.

Page 102: "Ura Koyama, 114; Reportedly World's 2nd-Oldest Person," *LA Times*, April 6, 2005

Page 105: 2005 Dietary Guidelines for Americans, United States Department of Health & Human Services

Page 111: *www.fitresource.com*.

Page 115: "Why it's hard to eat well and be active in America today," Center for Science in the Public Interest.

Page 118: "Statistics Related to Overweight and Obesity," National Institute of Diabetes and Digestive and Kidney Diseases, Weight-control Information Network.

Page 120: *www.diabetes.about.com*

Page 125: *www.fitresource.com*.

Page 135: "Obesity Surgery," American Obesity Association, AOA Advisor.

Page 137: "Magic Pill for Dieting? Wait for It on the Treadmill"; *The New York Times*, Tuesday, July 26, 2005, page F7.

Page 139: "Blood Sugar Problems Found After Weight-Loss Operation," *The New York Times*, Tuesday, July 26, 2005, page F7.

Page 141: "Slender Forever," *AARP The Magazine*, Volume 48, Number 5A, September-October 2005, page 20.

Page 143: "Obesity Surgery," American Obesity Association, AOA Advisor.

Page 145: "Homemade Dessert Disappearing From the Dinner Table," NPD Foodworld, September 16, 2003.

Page 150: "Dr. Phil's Fat Fighting Secrets," *Good Housekeeping*, August 2005, page 120.

Page 151: "Obesity in Youth," American Obesity Association, AOA Fact Sheets.

Page 153: "Stick to Your Diet This Holiday Season, WebMD tips for dieters on most popular diet plans" by Denise Mann, WebMD.

Page 156: "Obesity in Youth," American Obesity Association, AOA Fact Sheets.

Page 159: "Overweight and Obesity: Frequently Asked Questions," Department of Health and Human Services, Centers for Disease Control and Prevention.

Page 160: "Don't Let Grandma's Well-Meaning Pleas Sabotage Your Diet," by Kathleen Doheny, *LA Times*, April 10, 2005.

Page 164: "Americans May Be Finding Balance in Their Eating Patterns," NPD Foodworld, October 13, 2004.

Page 164: "Eating at Fast-food Restaurants More than Twice Per Week is Associated with More Weight Gain and Insulin Resistance in Otherwise Healthy Young Adults," *NIH News*, National Institutes.of Health, December 30, 2004.

Page 165: "The Food and Drug Administration's (FDA) Obesity Working Group Report," U.S. Food and Drug Administration, Center for Food Safety and Applied Nutrition.

Page 167: "From Wallet to Waistline: The Hidden Costs of Super Sizing," National Alliance for Nutrition and Activity.

Page 167: "The Contribution of Expanding Portion Sizes to the US Obesity Epidemic," by Lisa R. Young, PhD, and Marion Nestle, PhD, MPH, *American Journal of Public Health*, February 2002, Vol. 92, No. 2.

Page 168: National Heart, Lung, and Blood Institute.

Page 168: "How to Take Your Diet on Vacation," The AAA Traveler's Companion, January 2003.

Page 169: "Chain Reaction," by Daniel Kadlec, *Time*, June 7, 2004.

Page 169: "Americans May Be Finding Balance in Their Eating Patterns," NPD Foodworld, October 13, 2004.

Page 170: "Survey Shows More Low-Fat and Vegetarian Choices Available at Top US Airports," The Physicians Committee for Responsible Medicine, November 15, 2004.

Page 174: "Choosing a Safe and Successful Weight-loss Program," Weight-control Information Network, National Institute of Diabetes and Digestive and Kidney Diseases.

Page 177: "Diet and Health: Recent Research Developments," Economic Research Service, United States Department of Agriculture.

Page 183: "The NPD's New Dieting Monitor Tracks America's Dieting Habits," NPD Foodworld, May 3, 2004.

Page 185: "10 Things to Do when Your Diet's Not That Into You" by Stephanie Allmon, Fort Worth *Star-Telegram*, June 20, 2005.

Page 197: "Obesity Treatment," American Obesity Association, AOA Fact Sheets.

Page 200: "The NPD's New Dieting Monitor Tracks America's Dieting Habits," NPD Foodworld, May 3, 2004.

# HELP YOUR FRIENDS SURVIVE!

Order extra copies of *How to Lose 9,000 Lbs. (or Less)*, or one of our other books.

Please send me:

_____ copies of *How to Lose 9,000 Lbs. (or Less)* (@$13.95)

_____ copies of *How to Survive Your Teenager* (@$13.95)

_____ copies of *How to Survive a Move* (@$13.95)

_____ copies of *How to Survive Your Marriage* (@$13.95)

_____ copies of *How to Survive Your Baby's First Year* (@$12.95)

_____ copies of *How to Survive Dating* (@$12.95)

_____ copies of *How to Survive Your Freshman Year* (@$12.95)

Please add $3.00 for shipping and handling for one book, and $1.00 for each additional book. Georgia residents add 4% sales tax. Kansas residents add 5.3% sales tax. Payment must accompany orders. Please allow 3 weeks for delivery.

My check for $_____ is enclosed.

Please charge my __ Visa __ MasterCard __ American Express

Name _____

Organization _____

Address _____

City/State/Zip _____

Phone _____E-mail _____

Credit card # _____

Exp. Date _____Signature _____

Please make checks payable to Hundreds of Heads Books, LLC

# HELP WRITE THE NEXT **Hundreds of Heads**™ SURVIVAL GUIDE!

*Tell us your story about a life experience, and what lesson you learned from it. If we use your story in one of our books, we'll send you a free copy. Use this card or visit* **www.hundredsofheads.com**.

## Here's my story/advice on surviving

❏ **A New Job** (years working:_____ profession/job:_____)

❏ **A Move** (# of times you've moved:_____) ❏ **A Diet** (# of lbs. lost in best diet: ____)

❏ **A Teenager** (ages/sexes of your children: _____)

❏ **Divorce** (# of times married: _____ # of times divorced:_____)

❏ _____ **Other topic** (you pick)

Name: _____City/State: _____

❏ Use my name ❏ Use my initials only ❏ Anonymous

(Note: Your entry in the book may also include city/state and the descriptive information above.)

_____
Signature

How should we contact you *(this will not be published or shared)*:

e-mail: _____ other: _____

Please fax to 212-937-2220 or mail to:

Hundreds of Heads Books, LLC
#230
2221 Peachtree Road, Suite D
Atlanta, Georgia 30309

**Your story/advice:**

# VISIT WWW.HUNDREDSOFHEADS.COM

Do you have something interesting to say about marriage, your in-laws, dieting, holding a job, or one of life's other challenges?

Help humanity—share your story!

 Get published in our next book!

 Find out about the upcoming titles in the HUNDREDS OF HEADS™ survival guide series!

 Read up-to-the-minute advice on many of life's challenges!

 Sign up to become an interviewer for one of the next HUNDREDS OF HEADS™ survival guides!

Visit www.hundredsofheads.com today!

## Other Books from HUNDREDS OF HEADS™ BOOKS

HOW TO SURVIVE YOUR FRESHMAN YEAR . . . by Hundreds of Sophomores, Juniors, and Seniors Who Did (and some things to avoid, from a few dropouts who didn't)™
(April 2004; ISBN 0-9746292-0-0)

HOW TO SURVIVE DATING . . . by Hundreds of Happy Singles Who Did (and some things to avoid, from a few broken hearts who didn't)™
(October 2004; ISBN 0-9746292-1-9)

HOW TO SURVIVE YOUR BABY'S FIRST YEAR . . . by Hundreds of Happy Parents Who Did (and some things to avoid, from a few who barely made it)™
(January 2005; ISBN 0-9746292-2-7)

HOW TO SURVIVE YOUR MARRIAGE . . . by Hundreds of Happy Couples Who Did (and some things to avoid, from a few ex-spouses who didn't)™
(February 2005; 0-9746292-4-3)

HOW TO SURVIVE A MOVE . . . by Hundreds of Happy Dwellers Who Did (and some things to avoid, from a few who haven't unpacked yet)™
(April 2005; 0-9746292-5-1)

HOW TO SURVIVE YOUR TEENAGER . . . by Hundreds of Still-Sane Parents Who Did (and some things to avoid, from a few whose kids drove them nuts)™
(May 2005; ISBN 0-9746292-3-5)

## ABOUT THE EDITORS

JOAN BUCHBINDER is a sports nutritionist and head coach of The Nutrition Coaches of Brookline, Massachusetts, specializing in the areas of sports nutrition, weight loss, health, and wellness. Joan has worked with the non-athlete as well as recreational, collegiate, olympic, and professional athletes. For 17 years she served as the team nutritionist for the world champion New England Patriots football team, including Super Bowls XXXVI and XXXVIII. She has worked with The Boston Bruins hockey team, and The New England Revolution soccer team, and has provided weight loss and nutrition education programs at major corporations, school systems, colleges and universities. Joan has served as a consulting nutritionist with the U.S. Olympic Committee's sports nutrition program.

JENNIFER BRIGHT REICH is a special editor and headhunter for the HUNDREDS OF HEADS Survival Guide series. With more than 10 years of book-publishing experience, she has contributed to more than 70 books, including the South Beach Diet series. She lives in Hellertown, Pennsylvania, with her husband and new baby.